The
Insomnia
Answer

A Personalized Program
for Identifying and Overcoming
the Three Types of Insomnia

PAUL GLOVINSKY, Ph.D.
and
ARTHUR SPIELMAN, Ph.D.

A PERIGEE BOOK

THE BERKLEY PUBLISHING GROUP
Published by the Penguin Group
Penguin Group (USA) Inc.
375 Hudson Street, New York, New York 10014, USA
Penguin Group (Canada), 90 Eglinton Avenue East, Suite 700, Toronto, Ontario M4P 2Y3, Canada
(a division of Pearson Penguin Canada Inc.)
Penguin Books Ltd., 80 Strand, London WC2R 0RL, England
Penguin Group Ireland, 25 St. Stephen's Green, Dublin 2, Ireland (a division of Penguin Books Ltd.)
Penguin Group (Australia), 250 Camberwell Road, Camberwell, Victoria 3124, Australia
(a division of Pearson Australia Group Pty. Ltd.)
Penguin Books India Pvt. Ltd., 11 Community Centre, Panchsheel Park, New Delhi—110 017, India
Penguin Group (NZ), cnr. Airborne and Rosedale Roads, Albany, Auckland 1310, New Zealand
(a division of Pearson New Zealand Ltd.)
Penguin Books (South Africa) (Pty.) Ltd., 24 Sturdee Avenue, Rosebank, Johannesburg 2196,
South Africa
Penguin Books Ltd., Registered Offices: 80 Strand, London WC2R 0RL, England

ISBN: 0-399-53230-7

PRINTING HISTORY
Perigee hardcover edition / January 2006

PERIGEE is a registered trademark of Penguin Group (USA) Inc.
The "P" design is a trademark belonging to Penguin Group (USA) Inc.

This book has been cataloged by the Library of Congress

PRINTED IN THE UNITED STATES OF AMERICA

10 9 8 7 6 5 4 3 2 1

DEDICATION

This book is dedicated to my family. My parents, Norman and Celia Glovinsky, remained steadfast in their encouragement as I pursued diverse interests with no convergence in sight. My sisters, Ellen Busch and Lisa Berman, never let a few intervening states get in the way of a good talk. My sons, Isaac, Henry, and Will, initially provided me with object lessons on the effects of sleep loss. However, while I've dallied in accumulating clinical material for this volume, they have matured into perceptive young men. I look forward to their works.

To my wife, Maureen McNeil, I can only say that despite all the support I've enjoyed, this book—and more, this sweet life—would not be without you. *PBG*

To my family—mother Sunny, wife Marlene, and sons Evan and David— I dedicate this book. Thanks, Momma, for your funny, sunny ways that have brightened all my days. My eldest son, Evan, talented musician, my bike riding partner, and kind soul, I thank you for giving me that extra chance to connect in a meaningful way. David, gifted athlete, my intellectual playmate, and so high-spirited, many thanks for sharing your exploits. Marlene, your virtues defy enumeration. Thank you for providing the steady hand, daily stories, and especially the ever-present humor we have all thrived on. Because of all of you, I count my blessings. *AJS*

ACKNOWLEDGMENTS

I'm often asked how I became a sleep specialist. Was I a poor sleeper myself? No, it was serendipity rather than sleeplessness that set my course. At Montefiore Hospital in the Bronx, where I was training in neuropsychology, I happened upon the Laboratory of Human Chronophysiology—a truly timeless place with no clocks, no windows from which to gauge the sun, no radio or live TV. Some of the male staffers arrived at work clean-shaven; others would appear in the morning with stubble suggesting a five o'clock shadow. Living free of all time cues for weeks, laboratory volunteers were helping Elliot Weitzman and his team trace the threads that stitched together sleep and wakefulness. I switched my area of concentration that day (or was it night?).

At Montefiore, I had the good fortune to work with Charles Pollak and Michael Thorpy when sleep medicine was in first bloom. The case conferences they led felt more like expeditions, so new was the field. There, too, I found Aaron Sher and Arthur Spielman, who have been my close colleagues and cherished friends for more than twenty-five years.

As befits one of the world's foremost sleep apnea experts, Aaron lives and breathes the subject of sleep. Amidst all his clinical demands, Aaron has managed to maintain a true scholar's sense of wonder. His influence is infused throughout this work.

Acknowledgments

Arthur has kindled devotion to the quest of understanding sleep and its disorders in an entire generation of specialists. I proudly count myself among them. The intellectual gusto he brings to the chase and the joy he spreads among his associates are renowned. I am especially pleased that our long collaboration, truly a labor of love, has now taken such accessible form.

I am also delighted to have found new colleagues in Mark Rea and Mariana Figueiro and to have embarked on research combining their insights with those of Art and Aaron.

Special thanks are due to Edith Grossman, whose incisive letter encouraging consideration of graduate work in psychology found a receptive reader in Deadhorse, Alaska, where I was working cold, black nights on the oil pipeline. At the City University of New York, I found professors whose teachings continue to inform my work: Steven Ellman had just co-edited *The Mind in Sleep* and led a seminar that introduced me to this personally resonant topic. Arthur Arkin had a gentle assurance that meshed perfectly with his interest in hypnosis. I. H. Paul offered an appealing model of psychotherapy that aims for understanding while avoiding presumption and prying.

This book assumed its form out of the struggles and successes of many individuals. Although their names have been changed and their stories meshed into composites, I have tried to remain true to their experience. It has been my privilege to work with these patients—several of whom have told me how pleased they are that their stories might now help others. I also wish to thank the staff of the Capital Region Sleep/Wake Disorders Center in Albany, New York, where much of this work was done.

Finally, thanks are due to my literary agent, Jim Levine, whose exhortations to engage the reader have hopefully held sway, and to my editor at Perigee, Michelle Howry, whose enthusiasm for this project was evident from the start. *PBG*

My introduction to sleep science and clinical psychology began with my first mentor, Professor Steve Ellman at the City College of New York. In 1968, Steve helped me make the transition from the "late '60s" into a dazzling world of ideas and laboratory research. It was my great good fortune to have started with such a superb role model.

My first job in the field was with Drs. Elliot Weitzman, Howard Roffwarg, and Charles Pollak at the inception of the Sleep-Wake Disorders Center at Montefiore Hospital. I am proud to say that these three wise men trained me in sleep disorders medicine. Many fine physicians and psychologists did a stint at Montefiore, such as Richard Ferber, Mark Pressman, Paul Saskin, Daniel Wagner, Wolfgang Schmidt-Nowara, Paul Glovinsky, and the current director, Michael Thorpy. I know I learned from them, and I hope that they feel likewise.

The research arm of the endeavor at Montefiore became a "national resource" with such distinguished investigators as Charles Czeisler, Timothy Monk, Richard Coleman, and Margaret Moline joining to help set up the Laboratory of Human Chronophysiology. With such an all-star lineup, clinically and scientifically, we helped create a new discipline in those heady days. The training I received from this group was invaluable, and I will not soon forget the human side of our relationships.

Over the years at Montefiore, City College, New York Methodist Hospital, and New York Presbyterian Hospital (Cornell), I have worked with many stimulating and challenging graduate students. I certainly benefited from the give and take. I'll mention again Mark

Pressman and Paul Saskin, who got me started in the mentoring business. I thank them now for their forbearance then. My thanks to other former students, Drs. Lauren Broch, Stuart Cantor, Michael Anderson, Saul Rothenberg, Girardin Jean-Louis, Jessica Mitchell, Armando Margulis, John Adler, Andrew Tucker, Paul D'Ambrosio, Deirdre Conroy, Becky Quatrucci, and Matt Ebben, who helped shape my ideas while they fashioned careers in sleep medicine. A special thanks to Chien-Ming Yang, a most talented and dedicated former student and now collaborator. I hope all my students derive that pleasure of recognition as they see in this book the reflection of the flesh-and-blood work we did together.

My appreciation goes to Drs. Gerard Lombardo, Arthur Kotch, Neil Kavey, David Oelberg, and the other fine professionals with whom I have worked. These directors of sleep disorders centers have run first-rate programs and encouraged freedom of expression that permitted my ideas to take root and bloom.

The formulations and techniques Paul and I have contributed over the years need to be seen within the context of a long line of others' work. A list of influences can never be completely satisfying, but we do want to mention the seminal work of Drs. Peter Hauri and Richard Bootzin. Among their many contributions, work on sleep hygiene and on the psychological mechanisms underlying insomnia stand out as demarcating the beginnings of a behavioral conceptualization of the disorder. Along with the field in general, we thank Charles Morin, who has brought the thinking process into insomnia models. In addition, he has tied together key features of psychological treatment and built up a raft of research results that has buoyed us all.

I want to thank my friends, who are fellow sleep disorders travelers. They have provided both the safe harbor and the thrills of adventure that are both so necessary for the soul. John Herman, Jon Sassin, Max Hirshkowitz, Steve Lamstein, and Suzan Jaffe have been my traveling companions toward a destination at best dimly reckoned.

What a joy it has been working with my long-time collaborator and friend, Dr. Paul Glovinsky, for more than twenty-five years. A renaissance man, you will get an inkling of his gravitas, breadth, and sensitivity when you read this book. His clinical wisdom is rivaled only by his writing eloquence. Many thanks, Paul. They don't come any better than you.

Finally, to the field of sleep medicine, which is filled with smart, good, and caring people. I am proud to have participated in the beginnings of a great endeavor. *AJS*

CONTENTS

Contents

PART 2

The ABCDEs of Sleep

Contents

Contents

Contents

How Can I Mend My Broken Sleep?

Being hit with insomnia is a lot like having your heart broken. You feel betrayed and sapped of vitality; what used to flow naturally and effortlessly is now agonizing.

If you visit your doctor, not much shows up on examination. A lovelorn heart still pumps away, somehow oblivious to the gaping hole it harbors. An insomniac brain tethered to a fancy monitor usually just registers as awake. Although you may be certain some switch is stuck in the "on" position, it doesn't show up on the scans.

Despite your clean bill of health, both heartsickness and sleeplessness *feel* as if they have changed you, irreversibly, to the core. You muddle through your days and dread the approach of night. Instead of attending to your work or to your children, your mind continually drifts back toward your plight. Advice emanates from friends, strangers, doctors, TV, books, and magazines, all well-meaning and aiming to set you right: "You should get out more at night"; "Maybe it's time for a vacation"; "Here, take this pill."

It's a fair bet that you've followed plenty of such advice, only to discover that it helps for just a little while, if at all. After enough dis-appointments, you've probably begun to lose faith you will ever be healed.

That's why we want to assure you at the outset that we have the experience to help you sleep again. We are both clinical psychologists and specialists in the evaluation and treatment of sleep disorders, each with more than twenty-five years of experience helping thousands of patients successfully overcome their insomnia. We are Diplomates of the American Board of Sleep Medicine and co-directors of Sleep Disorders Centers accredited by the American Academy of Sleep Medicine. And we constructed what has become a standard developmental model of insomnia, one that is now regularly taught to aspiring sleep specialists around the world. Although we have explained the workings of this model many times to professionals and to our patients, this book contains its first presentation to readers who are suffering with insomnia.

The Insomnia Answer

Regardless of the type of insomnia you are contending with, we can help you improve your sleep. We will show you how to achieve more restful sleep—even if you have already followed sound sleep hygiene recommendations, such as cutting back on caffeine or avoiding daytime naps. We can help even if your insomnia has defied the purchase of a fancy new mattress, grueling gym workouts, Valerian tea at bedtime, or the latest hypnotic medication.

Insomnia can act like quicksand—the harder you try to climb out of its grasp, the deeper you become mired. Almost every remedy works on occasion, sometimes even for a few nights in a row. Just when you're thinking you've found the answer, however, sleep re-fuses to play along. Your brain is somehow able to resist both modern psychopharmacology and traditional folk wisdom and cling to its sleepless ways.

Given this kind of experience, we wouldn't blame you for feeling skeptical about our therapeutic claims. What are we offering that you haven't already tried? The answer may be surprising—although perhaps not to those who know how to respond when engulfed in quicksand: we will show you how to *be still* when unable to sleep, still in both body and mind. We will teach you how to *stop trying* to sleep, and instead rely on scientific principles to *position* yourself for sleep, just as a surfer catches a wave. We will help you *change atti-tudes and behaviors* that, although developed in response to insom-nia, only serve to perpetuate it.

We will start by exploring how *thinking* about sleep affects your ability to achieve that state. After enough experience with sleeplessness, sleeping ceases to be a "no-brainer"—a state that au-tomatically follows a period of wakefulness. Instead, it becomes something to dwell on and worry about—a performance issue. Doubts and anxieties trick your mind into becoming its own sabo-teur: you may think you long for sleep with all your might, yet some small, unruly part of your brain still manages to mount a successful resistance against that objective. We will show you how to detach yourself from sleep, how to stop striving for it and straining against it at the same time.

Second, we will apply newfound scientific insights to help you position yourself for sleep. Our program is based on a model of circadian rhythms developed and refined in research labs over the last twenty years but not yet widely known to the general public. We integrate this newly discovered understanding of the *physiology of*

3

sleep with a comprehensive approach to the *psychology of sleep* that will orient both your body and mind toward a restful night.

As we will explain more fully throughout this book, sleep/wake cycles roll through our minds and bodies like ocean waves. You can sleep better by learning to catch these waves. And it doesn't matter what the source of your sleep problems are: childhood trauma, pain or discomfort caused by a medical condition, worries, personality traits, or life's stresses. When you understand and appreciate how your body balances its drive for sleep with an opposing force for alertness and how your mind can either invite sleep or resist it, you will begin to feel that sleeping well is possible again.

Third, we will show you how to distinguish the factors that led to your sleep problem from those that are maintaining it. This is not some dry academic exercise, but essential to getting you back to sleep. Targeting the right problems can improve sleep with surprising speed, while at the same time helping you avoid months or years of fruitless effort. You may be surprised to learn that sometimes the experience that *triggers* insomnia (salient or even traumatic as that experience may be) is *not* the best place to intervene therapeutically.

Even as we bring all our personal experience and collective knowledge to bear on your problem, we would not be confident of success if we did not have access to a key resource: we're speaking of *you*, acting as our colleague. Insomnia is a tricky business. Sleeplessness can behave in a totally opposite manner from one individual to another. Some insomniacs, for example, have more trouble sleeping in a hotel room than they do at home. Others actually sleep better when their surroundings are unfamiliar because their own bedrooms have become so thoroughly associated with poor sleep. Some insomniacs wear earplugs to block out as much noise as possible as they await sleep. But others keep a radio turned to a low volume because they are comforted by a bit of background patter to keep them company.

So when it comes to changing the way *you* sleep, we will need to consult with the world's reigning expert on the matter. You are the one who best knows the history of your sleep disturbance, who can ferret out clues to its onset, and who can reconstruct scenes where sleep miraculously appeared. You are the one who is most familiar with details of your daily life, bedtime rituals, and nighttime struggles. This book will be supplying the questions—asking how you think about your sleep, how you behave regarding your sleep or your sleeplessness, what changes you might consider, and what interventions you might wish to try. You, however, will be supplying the answers.

When You Need Sleep *Tonight*

Some of you may be groaning. "This is too much—it will take too long! Can't you just tell me what to do—or better yet, what to take—so my sleep is better tonight? I'm exhausted and desperate. I can't take another night without sleep!"

Fair enough. There are instances when getting more sleep right away makes a lot of sense, whether because you are forced to deal with an ongoing crisis, in mourning, or trying to avert a psychological meltdown. If you feel you belong in this group, you should talk to your physician before proceeding much further with this book. In such emergencies, medication is often indicated for at least short-term use, be it a sleeping pill or of another type. After your situation has stabilized, you will be ready to join in our collaboration toward a long-term solution to your problem.

From the rest of you—especially those with a small pharmacy of sleep aids already squirreled away in your medicine cabinet, those who draw from an array of over-the-counter and prescription medications, mixing and matching, breaking off small pieces of the stronger stuff for later in the night or to stretch your supply—we are asking for a few weeks. Not to become "former insomniacs"—we'll state up front that for many of you, that achievement will be a long-term goal. No, we will need a few weeks just to convince you that *you are able to influence your sleep*, that your seemingly random sleep pattern indeed has rhyme and reason—that it in fact *responds* to rhyme and to reason.

In the meantime, if you are taking sleeping pills on the recommendation of your physician, stick to what has been prescribed for you. We will be able to work together and put changes into effect that will ultimately enhance your ability to sleep naturally while you continue on your medicine. When you are beginning to see improvement and feeling more confident in your ability to sleep, we will encourage you to speak with your doctor about a plan for gradually tapering your reliance on pills.

Give This Plan Time

Having just bargained for a few weeks, some words on the healing power of time are in order. When most people (that is, those who are not destined to become chronic insomniacs) suffer from sleeplessness, their first-line treatment is simply the passage of time. Most cases of transient insomnia remain just that—transient. They run their course as time passes and are gone. Exactly how does time act as a balm? Perhaps more to the point for our discussion, why is it that time is not *always* a balm? It is instructive here to hearken back to our opening analogy, which likened insomnia to heartache.

Time is the treatment most often recommended to heal a broken heart. Its active ingredients are the thousand and one little intrusions daily life contains. Consider the following scenario: heartbroken, you've slept late, moped around the house, and skipped both breakfast and lunch. Eventually, hunger catches up with you, and you realize that you don't even have any junk food in the cupboard for dinner. You drag yourself out of the house, eyes fixed on the sidewalk as you slouch toward the corner store. By the entrance, you glance at an advertisement for an upcoming movie. "They're forever making sequels" you mutter to yourself, but then you can't quite suppress a smile as you recall a scene from the original picture. Making your way to the frozen foods section, you realize with a start that you have actually spent the last minute or two thinking about this film. Unbelievable as it sounds, you were distracted from your suffering by a movie poster!

Through such small incursions, pain is gradually replaced by numbness, or at least edged out by trivia. Daily experience is indifferent to your plight, and it bombards you mercilessly. Small moments of distraction clump together, eventually swaddling your heart. Thus protected from fresh pain, you can finally begin to heal. There may be a residual scar or two, but your capacity to trust and to love again is more or less restored.

A similar healing process usually occurs over time when sleep is disrupted. Think now of how a generally "good sleeper" might react to a poor night of sleep. She might indeed feel awful as the alarm clock finally rings, but soon after arising, she is already getting pulled into the morning rush. Sleeplessness may have loomed large in a darkened bedroom at three in the morning, but by the light of day, its irksome consequences are manageable. When a jarring phone call is received mid-day, our good sleeper mobilizes to meet the challenge. The trials of the night just past are now far from her mind. If she thinks of sleep at all, it might be to relish the prospect of getting into bed again, knowing from past experience that a particularly deep and satisfying night of sleep awaits her.

Unfortunately, time does not always work such wonders. Once insomnia becomes established, it can be fueled rather than quieted by nightly encounters with bed. If you have reached this state, where your sleeplessness has only worsened with the passage of time, where each night brings fresh rebuff to your attempts at sleep, where you now doubt your ability to ever sleep well again, we invite you to get out of bed and work with us. We will be asking you to make all kinds of changes in your behavior shortly. But for now, we ask only that you begin to think about sleep anew.

New thinking is the key to our program. Don't worry, we're not about to cram your head with facts. A stream of facts might put people to sleep in a lecture hall, but we have found that they are really not that useful for people contending with insomnia. What works better is the *reassurance that comes with understanding*. You will soon gain a new understanding of sleep, and in particular, of why you are not sleeping well. You will come to appreciate that your mind, now a source of strife in bed, can actually be a good partner when it comes to finding sweet dreams.

PART ONE

Catching the
Wave of Sleep

By the time you seek help for insomnia, it's likely that you know a lot about sleep, at least insofar as your own is concerned. You've had a lot of time to think things over as you've waited out the night, passing the time until morning confirms that you've been stood up again. One conclusion you've probably come to is that sleep cannot be trusted. Sleep seems to play by its own rules—or perhaps no rules at all. It mocks your efforts to be conscientious to the point where you have likely given up and decided to do whatever it takes to bring yourself some relief. That might mean using sleeping pills, spending half the night on the Internet, sleeping into the morning, relying on coffee to get through the afternoon, or a host of other strategies.

These strategies are not without their own drawbacks, but they are the best you've been able to come up with after years of trial and error, and they have enabled you to muddle through to this point. You would be understandably wary of anyone who proposes that you abandon or even modify them. After all, you're the one who has to pull yourself out of bed each morning, with whatever sleep you have managed to accumulate, and face the day. At the very least, you'd want to be sure your would-be benefactor could provide a convincing rationale for any proposed changes in the way you tackle your problem.

That is exactly what we propose to do in Part 1 of this book. We appreciate that your responses to chronic insomnia, whether mental or physical, are entrenched for good reason. You've had your fill of directives, suggestions, and tips. Before we dare add to the list, we hope to impart something else—a working knowledge of sleep and insomnia as currently understood by clinicians and researchers, to complement and perhaps challenge your personal convictions.

We start in Chapter 1 by examining a question that is fundamental yet rarely asked: why is sleep so unreliable? That sleep is crucial to health, efficiency, and safety has been the take-home message of recent research. We are learning more each year how illnesses, losses in productivity, and accidents are brought on when we voluntarily cut short sleep or follow irregular sleep/wake schedules. Given this central role for sleep, how is it possible that so many of us experience insomnia in our quiet and safe bedrooms, despite our fervent wish to sleep?

In exploring this key question, we will come to see that far from being an aberration, sleeplessness seems to be a by-product of our evolution. Physically, we are more prone to arousal than to sleep. Starting from a placid state, we can become agitated in seconds, whereas it may take us hours to fully calm down. Our mental functioning also tilts toward wakefulness: To the extent that we employ foresight to anticipate threats, we put our own sleep at risk. In a hypochondriac's nightmare, the mere inkling that insomnia might occur can be sufficient to bring it on.

Fortunately, thoughtfulness has also provided us with scientific understanding that can help redress this imbalance. In Chapter 2, we present a schematic explanation of how sleep is supposed to happen—how, under ideal conditions, sleep and wakefulness are organized into waves. This formulation is quite counterintuitive. It suggests that, even though we experience levels of arousal along a single dimension ranging from deep sleep through full alertness, this arousal actually results from the blending of *two* distinct forces. We call these the Sleep Drive and the Alerting Force. They are regulated by different physiological mechanisms and can either work in concert to produce a well-defined sleep/wake cycle or get in each other's way to yield sleep that sputters out in dribs and drabs.

In Chapter 3, we consider the specific ways in which sleep can go wrong. We pose a question that may have circled round your head at night: "How did I get insomnia?" To answer this question, we present a developmental model of insomnia that separates contributing factors into three groups: (1) inherited or acquired characteristics that raise the risk of insomnia; (2) events, ranging from the cataclysmic to the mundane, that trigger the onset of insomnia; and (3) attitudes, beliefs, and behaviors that maintain insomnia after it has become established. Understanding this model is clinically useful because it directs attention toward the factors underlying your sleeplessness that are most easily treated. It should give hope to those of you who can trace the onset of your insomnia to specific past events that now seem beyond therapeutic reach. And it will also help those who are bewildered by the lack of any clear-cut starting point for their sleep disturbance.

At the outset of our discussion we stressed how, for better or for worse, thinking is critical to sleep. Hours of sleeplessness can be triggered by what would have otherwise been a fleeting thought. Over the long run, the specific attitudes we harbor about sleep go a long way in determining how restful our nights will be. The *value* placed on sleep is also important—sleep does best when it is neither discounted nor too highly prized. In Chapter 4, we ask that you consider what sleep means for you. We also request that you examine your feelings about easing your vigilance, tuning out your inner voice, and relinquishing control over your consciousness. As you learn to unmoor yourself from the contents of your mind and float over your thoughts, you will be much better positioned to catch the Wave of Sleep.

CHAPTER ONE

Why Is Sleep So Unreliable?

Discovering Why Sleep Doesn't Come Naturally

Adam lay expectantly on his newly laundered sheet, his wife sleeping quietly not one foot away. Everything was in order: he was fresh from a shower; the briefcase on his desk was emptied of files; he could sense a wave of sleepiness approaching.

The sounds outside the window were reassuring. The late stragglers on the sidewalk, the traffic noise, the hum of the air conditioners—all meshed into a soothing blend. Adam knew his sleep required such a harmonious context, and he took pains to provide it. He glanced with envy at Jen, who laughed at his precautions, and who was known to fall asleep on buses, on sofa beds, even once at the ball game.

Adam tried to rein in his thoughts, but they drifted toward the presentation he had to make the next afternoon. If this happened to be one of his bad nights, he would really be out of sorts by two o'clock. He could feel his muscles tighten at the thought. Adam loosened his jaw the way he'd been taught and tried to slow down his breathing.

He had grown quite competent at hiding the effects of his sleeplessness. Sometimes he would play the stolid manager, unperturbed by the most harrowing crises. Other times he would slip into hyperactive mode, keeping himself awake by keeping everyone else hopping. But a presentation to the parent company could not be finessed so easily. Adam became aware of his increased heart rate. He could no longer pretend that nothing was wrong. Perhaps tomorrow would be the day when, sleep-deprived, his fumbles and miscues would alert senior management to his real predicament: on a fundamental level, he was out of control.

This was going to be a long night.

How is it that so many of us cannot readily fall asleep or stay asleep? After all, sleep is inborn, a state attained in infancy without any instruction or practice. It should be automatic.

We may eat too much or too little, but almost all of us *are able to eat* when food is available. Unless we are contending with serious medical illness, we all take breathing in and out for granted. Insomnia, by contrast, is widespread in otherwise healthy people. In its intermittent, acute form, it is familiar to practically everyone. As a chronic sleep disorder, it afflicts 10 to 15 percent of the population. How can something so crucial to normal functioning be so unreliable? And how is it that some people require everything to be just right before they can sleep, while others seem to be able to drop off at will?

These are questions that may come to you in the middle of the night, as you watch the glowing red lines on your alarm clock. Your dog snoring away on the rug seems to be able to sleep on cue. He circles into bed every evening as darkness gathers, and soon afterward seems to be chasing dream squirrels. Sleepy animals outside your home also find their havens and perches by nightfall, while the nocturnal ones begin to stir, all according to schedule. Even most of your human neighbors are sleeping—despite whatever might be on their minds. It all looks so easy, so natural. Why can't you sleep?

Your question is straightforward, but unfortunately, its answer is not. When your car won't move, the fact that you can describe the problem succinctly doesn't mean its solution will be self-evident. To get on the road again, you might run through a simple checklist: *Is there gas in the tank? Is the battery dead? Do I need to find a mechanic?* In other words, to solve your problem, you would have to know something—either a little or a lot—about cars.

This analogy holds true for sleep as well. A checklist to consult if your sleep has stalled *does* exist. It is called a list of Sleep Hygiene Instructions. We assume that most of you will be familiar with these recommendations—although whether you can actually adhere to them is another question! It makes sense to review this list before proceeding, because it just might supply a direct fix for your sleep. In the course of our work together, you will come to understand how these sleep hygiene prescriptions enhance your prospects for sleep. For now, our advice would be to simply be sure you are following them—if your sleep starts running smoothly, you can then read on and learn why at your leisure!

Sleep Hygiene Instructions

❑ **Avoid going to bed until you are drowsy.** Maintain a consistent rising time, even if you go to bed late, whether during the workweek or on weekends.

❑ **Limit napping.** If you must take a nap, it should be short—about half an hour—and finished by mid-afternoon.

- ❑ Avoid all caffeine after noon. Limiting yourself to one cup in the morning is best.

- ❑ Avoid nicotine and alcohol in the evening, or if you awaken at night.

- ❑ Avoid exercising in the late evening, or if you awaken at night. Vigorous exercise ending four to six hours before bedtime, on the other hand, may deepen your sleep.

- ❑ Limit fluids as much as possible in the four to six hours before bedtime.

- ❑ Be sure your bedroom is dark, quiet, and well ventilated. Keep it at a comfortable temperature. Turn your clock so you cannot read the time if you awaken at night. Be sure your pet is not disturbing your sleep.

We understand that these prescriptions are deceptively straightforward. It's easy enough to pledge to "Limit napping," for example, but much harder in practice to pass up the opportunity to catch up on sleep for an hour or two after a particularly rough night. If your sleep does not improve following reasonable compliance with these instructions, do not despair. We have written this book with you in mind. We won't pretend that it will make you a full-fledged sleep specialist. But you should be able to perform tune-ups and basic repairs. Let's get started with a discussion of why something as fundamental as sleep can nonetheless be so unreliable. You will soon learn that the apparent simplicity of sleep is also deceptive—its appearance actually depends upon the coordination of a complex array of factors. Moreover, some of the key attributes that differentiate our species from other animals also predispose us to sleeplessness. In effect, insomnia is all too human!

Sleep Is Complicated

Sleep used to be thought of as a kind of backdrop—a dark, inert curtain against which our waking lives played out. We believed sleep simply appeared by default whenever alertness waned. But after more than fifty years of research, we can decisively reject this lifeless view of sleep. Sleep is actively produced by subcortical brain mechanisms. Its structure (known as its *architecture*) reflects a three-way parlay among competing interests: the body's requirement for deeper, quieter *Non-Rapid Eye Movement* (*NREM*) *sleep*; intermittent need for more physiologically active and cognitively stimulating *Rapid Eye Movement* (*REM*) *sleep;* and a fluctuating propensity to be *awake.* The result of such internal negotiation is a cyclic alternation of NREM and REM sleep stages occurring about every ninety minutes, with the deepest NREM sleep stages, known as *Slow Wave Sleep*, taking precedence in the initial cycles and REM sleep gaining ascendancy later in the night. Ideally, five or so NREM/REM cycles provide us with about eight hours of sleep, after which we should awaken refreshed for the day ahead.

The complexity of sleep goes beyond its structure. Sleep is

- a *physical* state, characterized by relative stillness and repose.

- a *mental* state, characterized by reduced arousal and lowered vigilance.

- motivated by a *physiological drive*—our craving for sleep grows stronger when we stay awake and is sated as we slumber.

- regulated by an *inner body clock* that orchestrates our internal workings while keeping us synchronized to the cycle of day and night.

- responsive to *behavior*—sleep is inhibited by activity and induced when we are sedentary.

- dependent upon finding an *appropriate environment.*

In all these ways, human sleep is similar to sleep found throughout most of the animal kingdom. Animals generally seek out safe havens and stop moving when they sleep, although there are surprising exceptions—such as the dolphins that sleep with half their brains at a time as they slowly circle on the water's surface. The timing of most animals' sleep is cyclic, with one major sleep period—whether during the night or day—aligned to the environmental light/dark cycle via the same biological clock we humans share. Again, there are exceptions, such as the repeated snoozes of your house cat, reflecting its predatory heritage.

Thinking Can Cause Insomnia

Human sleep has evolved along these general outlines, but it does not adhere to them rigidly. If it did, getting to sleep would be simply a matter of finding the right time and the right place. Unfortunately, our vaunted ability to plan ahead, borne of a highly developed forebrain, has had the side effect of greatly expanding the range of circumstances deemed inappropriate for sleep. So even when snug in bed on a tranquil night, we are still able to *anticipate* or *imagine* threats that can forestall sleep as surely as would a real wolf at the door.

Sleep, then, depends upon cooperation from the environment, the body, and the mind. The clanging of road construction, a sore hip, or financial worries are each sufficient to waylay its appearance. The prospects for sleep are even more dicey than these prerequisites would suggest, in that the environment, body, and mind *interact*. The challenge is like that faced by a mother of triplets, who must strive to keep all three children content simultaneously because the howls of one can easily set off the others.

Let's observe this interaction in practice. Suppose you have just moved into a new apartment and realize, as you lay wide awake in the dark, that your bed is situated directly beneath your upstairs neighbor's media room. Your sleep will soon be under attack on all fronts: your ears register booming bass soundwaves that by themselves would make sleep unlikely, your muscles tense with each rumble, and your heart rate quickens. At this point, your sleep already has two strikes against it—both the environment and your body are dissenting. Finally, your mind lodges *its* protest, as you berate yourself for not checking with the previous tenant about the action-film buff upstairs, and start hatching soundproofing schemes or ways to escape your lease. At this point, your prospects for sleep are quite remote—even when your neighbor finally finishes watching his movie and turns in for the night.

• • •

Now we can begin to see why sleep appears more reliably for your dog than for you. Both you and Snuggles require a reasonably full belly, as well as other creature comforts, to slumber. Both of you are regulated by the rising and setting sun—to a degree, we shall see, that you may find surprising. You both need to feel a sense of security. It's just that you, with your higher brain functions, are much more exacting when it comes to granting yourself a safe passage into sleep. To be sure, sometimes having a big brain helps ease the way. You may sleep through a thunderstorm while your dog whimpers under the bed because you can reason that the storm *sounds* more menacing than it actually is. More often, however, your pet's limited risk assessment, which does not take into account such factors as bothersome neighbors, factory closings, or the approach of tax deadlines, will result in an evaluation more conducive to sleep.

Insomnia Can Be Learned or Innate

The relative contribution of "nature" versus "nurture" in determining human behavioral patterns is a perennial source of debate among academics. It is safe to say that in recent years the role of "nature," as represented by genetic inheritance, has loomed large in both actual discoveries and the popular imagination. Psychiatric illnesses and behavioral disorders that were at one time thought to result primarily from a given familial or social context are now known to stem at least in part from genetic predispositions, sometimes located to specific genes. The once-derided excuse "I was born that way" is not now so easily dismissed.

However, the presence or absence of a particular genetic endowment is usually not enough to accurately predict the onset of illness. Much of the time, theorists end up constructing more complicated models to explain the appearance of a given disorder. They may suggest, for example, a latent genetic predisposition, which is then activated by environmental factors. Insomnia is just now beginning to be appreciated along such lines. It has long been understood that "nurture," in the form of both routine and traumatic experience, can lead to sleep problems. More recently, sleep specialists have focused their attention on "nature," that is, on inborn characteristics that predispose some individuals to sleep well and others toward sleeplessness.

> Karla was towed into the consultation behind her weary and exasperated mother. She had always been a "poor sleeper." Karla's mother recalled how, during her first years of life, she never slept more than an hour or two at a time. Other children in her toddler group would nap on cue when their little mats were rolled out and konk out again as soon as they began the drive home, but Karla would alternate between perkiness and irritability rather than between wakefulness and sleep.
>
> Now four years old, Karla never just fell asleep—rather, she would collapse out of exhaustion. Peace would then reign for a few hours. Around midnight, Karla would rouse with a wail and require an elaborate soothing routine before succumbing to sleep once more. She awoke again around five in the morning, when her screams would effectively end the night for her parents. Her mother smiled as she marveled at how Karla's older sister, cocooned not five feet away, would somehow manage to sleep unperturbed through each night's saga.

While some of you may find this hard to believe, all of us inherit at least some propensity to fall asleep, in addition to a tendency to become aroused. Sleep mechanisms have been preserved and refined over the course of evolution, presumably because sleep served a number of adaptive functions for our ancestors. These roles may have been as disparate as energy conservation, strengthening the immune system, or protection from predators, yet they shared the common outcome of promoting survival. Just as height distributes normally in the population—with most people near an average height and fewer at either extreme—so, too, there are innate differences in the strength of the sleep drive and in the level of wakefulness that supports our daily functioning.

Recent research points to the conclusion that chronically heightened levels of wakefulness may represent a *trait*, a relatively stable characteristic that is shared by a large percentage of people contending with chronic insomnia. This trait is termed *hyperarousal*. People with this trait will, for example, secrete higher levels of *adrenocorticotropic hormone* from the pituitary gland or *cortisol* from the adrenal gland in a stressful situation, which in turn will lead to higher levels of activation. Hyperarousal in insomnia is also manifest in a higher metabolic rate, which can be detected by an increased body temperature using elaborate sensors. As with other traits, the tendency toward hyperarousal has likely been shaped by evolutionary pressures. Evidently, this trait has also been advantageous to survival, as it is so widespread today!

As sleep specialists advance their understanding of the inheritance of sleep patterns, they are catching up with common knowledge. Parents of two or more children are often amazed at how early differences in sleep propensity are evident in their offspring. They will be rightly skeptical of explanations that attribute these differences solely to child-rearing practices that shift from one child to the next: good or poor sleep, they will recall, was apparent from the first days and weeks of postnatal life (or perhaps even in the womb!)—presumably before their parenting styles could have had much impact. Of course, once differing patterns of sleep are established, parents will doubtless begin to respond to their children in different ways—a critically important factor in reinforcing these patterns.

In any insomnia support group, the contributions of both "nature" and "nurture" are readily apparent. Some in the group can pinpoint the night their sleep problems started, linked to an explicit trigger such as illness, divorce, or financial disaster. Others might not be able to say exactly when their insomnia had its onset, but they can recall fourteen, thirty-two, or even sixty-eight years of reasonably satisfying sleep before things began to fall apart.

The most hardened insomniacs in the group (and their parents, if asked!) will attest that, like Karla, they have not slept well from the day they were born. Times might be stressful or carefree, the bed might be sagging or comfortable, they could be nursing a shoulder injury or in the best of health—it would hardly matter insofar as their poor sleep was concerned. These sleepless souls are walking evidence for the contribution of "nature" in instigating insomnia. A special diagnostic category—*idiopathic insomnia*—has been reserved to denote the innate, primary, and chronic sleep disturbance with which they struggle.

Socialization Can Cause Insomnia

Our earliest sleep/wake schedules are largely unfettered by social constraints. As babies, we sleep when we are comfortable, when there is nothing particularly stimulating going on, when we have been awake for a while. We sleep to grow, to replenish the energy-consuming processes of development that were so recently humming along in the womb.

This blissful freedom does not last long. Unbeknownst to us, our self-selected sleep schedules have a great impact on our parents, as they struggle to accommodate our needs in the middle of the night. We begin to receive training in how to sleep—or more precisely, in when to fall asleep and in how long to sleep. It is at this point that the central fact regarding sleep that we have been discussing becomes evident: we all vary in our ability to fall asleep at a given time, in our ability to stay asleep, and in how much sleep we seem to need. Some of us can sleep through a raging thunderstorm, and others are awakened by a faucet drip. This natural variation in sleep propensity leads us to be tagged by exhausted parents with one of our very first evaluations: we are either esteemed as "good sleepers" or else bemoaned as "up all night long." Sleep has become an issue of performance. Although the initial venue for this performance is the crib, the same demands may persist right through adulthood, as we struggle in bed to meet academic and workplace schedules.

Regardless of exactly how we came to sleep well or poorly, we soon know where we lie on the issue. Sleep has become woven into our self-image, providing a flash point for anxiety. Before long, we do not need our parents or anyone else to rate us—we learn to judge for ourselves how well we can sleep. If sleep has not presented much of a problem, we may not give it much thought or even think of it as a natural rhythm akin to respiration. If we have struggled with sleep, we will learn to label ourselves as "insomniacs," look upon sleep to be about as intuitive as tightrope walking, and devote much mental and physical energy to the task of attaining it.

Sleep Is a Risk

We have seen that the relative balance between sleepiness and wakefulness varies among individuals. However, considering human beings as a species, wakefulness takes precedence. There are good reasons behind our tendency to favor consciousness. While sleep has apparently been critical to evolutionary success, as might be inferred from its preservation across the animal kingdom, in the short run, sleeping may put us at risk. On the scale of daily life, it is consciousness—and in particular, vigilance—that is adaptive. Out in the field, only those predators at the top of the food chain, such as lions, might devour half a zebra and then settle down into an unconcerned snooze. The other links in the chain were eventually shaped to become pickier about sleep.

Even though we humans have schemed our way to a dominant position in modern times, the brainstem mechanisms that regulate our sleep evolved under more precarious circumstances, and they are wired accordingly: we are tilted toward wakefulness—quick to arouse and slow to calm down. Our physiology supports this bias. Faced with a challenge, our heart rate quickens and our muscles tense. We are geared for action, not sleep. We preserve enough of our wits about us, even when sleep-deprived, to be able to choose between "fight or flight." We wait for an unambiguous "all-clear" signal before allowing ourselves to sleep. Of course, we can only keep up our guard so long before eventually succumbing to exhaustion. Many of you will recognize this sequence as the pattern of your own sleep—long stretches of sleeplessness or broken sleep, followed by complete collapse.

Thus, sleep in human adults is facing a two-strike count. First, we still appear to be sleeping the sleep of the hunted, not of the hunter. We are adept at rallying our attention and maintaining a vigil against threats, but less capable when it comes to settling ourselves down. Second, having gained our ascendant position in the food chain through executive functioning as opposed to larger teeth or more powerful limbs, having learned to fashion secure homes with locked doors while confining most of our erstwhile enemies to zoos, we are now saddled with brains that got where they are in large measure *by not sleeping* and that are primed to respond to new threats at a moment's notice. Unfortunately, our modern world provides myriad threats, all capable of disrupting sleep—from burglars to bankruptcy, from social snubs to terrorism.

A major task facing the sleepy brain, therefore, becomes one of gauging just how appropriate it is to sleep. In former days, this was a fairly straightforward procedure, centered primarily on physical safety. Even in modern societies, many people still contend with safety concerns on a nightly basis. Then there are those who may be physically secure but jockeying for comfort and quiet among a host of siblings or other relatives. The luckiest have their own comfortable beds in their own rooms. What's left to get in the way of sleep for them, one might ask? The answer is plenty. Threats to sleep still lurk in the form of academic deadlines, unresolved arguments, sales quotas, upcoming social events, and other pressures of modern life. The body can feel comfortable and secure, but the mind may still judge conditions too uncertain to sleep.

As long as these threats to sleep are external, sleep can be protected by meeting one's challenges head-on during waking hours. The student facing a deadline can buckle down and begin writing the paper; the salesperson can schedule additional calls with potential customers. Sleep can also be protected by minimizing the threat, at least in one's mind, or by looking the other way. The student can determine that his paper might be written tomorrow afternoon; the salesperson can assume that her poor numbers will be buried in the monthly report. No matter how dire an external menace looms, we can take comfort in the knowledge that our sleep will return once the crisis is resolved. Oftentimes, just that realization can be enough to allow ourselves off the hook. We'll "deal with it in the morning."

A critical juncture is passed, however, when the threat to sleep is perceived as internal. If we begin to think that we are physiologically incapable of sleeping well, or that we cannot turn off our minds, we will have fallen under the sway of an omnipresent threat, one that we carry within ourselves, portaged from night to night. At this point, we have created an insomnia that can feed itself—a sleep disturbance that can survive even when our daily lives are relatively trouble-free. Sleep itself has become the problem, and it begins to consume much of our waking thoughts. It ceases to be unremarkable. As sleep becomes more meaningful, it also becomes more elusive.

Sleep Is Out of Your Control

If sleep is so fugitive—if it vanishes in the face of real threats, perceived threats, even the *thought* of a threat—how can you ever hope to rely on it? If it can slip out of your grasp like water, how can we be so sure you will be sleeping well again? The answer to this critical question is in fact suggested by water. The waves of the sea are also beyond your control, beyond your grasp. But this does not mean you cannot learn to swim, to surf, to sail a boat, or even, with enough ingenuity and expense, to harness the tides. Key to all these marine pursuits is an understanding of water and submission to its nature.

In each case, fighting the waves will prove hopeless, whereas those who literally "go with the flow" will meet with success.

So it is with sleep. You have no doubt convinced yourself by sorry experience that you can no more command sleep to appear than you can part the waves. Even the most meticulous and controlling of you will, like Adam—the manager we met at the start of this chapter—have met your match. To sleep well again, you will need to *work with sleep rather than against it.* Just as the fledgling swimmer must at some point relax and trust in the power of buoyancy, you, too, will learn to let yourself be carried off by sleep. And just as the experienced surfer gauges where and when to catch the perfect wave, you, too, will learn to gracefully ride the sleep/wake cycle.

In the next chapter, we introduce you to the physiological dynamics that generate waves of sleep. While you may find the diagrams you encounter there intimidating, we will be at your side, explaining each step. Stay with us. Whether you achieve a comprehensive grasp of the mechanics of sleep and wakefulness or only the general idea, your efforts at understanding will be amply rewarded as we set you on the course toward more reliable and restful sleep.

CHAPTER TWO

How Is Sleep Supposed to Happen?

Building a Wave of Sleep

Fran glanced at her watch and bemoaned the long day ahead. It was just ten o'clock, and she had already been up for nearly seven hours! After work, she was supposed to meet her mother for a birthday dinner and then stay awake through an entire program of English composers. Her first thought was that it just couldn't be done—she would have to bail out. Fran tried to recall the excuses she had resorted to most recently, not wanting to overplay the list. She realized with a start that her kids must seem quite sickly to her family and friends by now. Perhaps she could wait until after lunch before making a decision.

By mid-afternoon, Fran's premonitions were confirmed. Swaying in her chair, her eyes refused to focus on the fresh marketing report posed on her desk, still turned to page three. *I'll never be able to stay out tonight*, she thought. *Getting through the day will be challenge enough.* Rallying her faculties, Fran tried to gauge the risks of resting her head on the spiral-bound sheaf and shutting her eyes for a few minutes. She had heard enough about the new management, though, to know that power napping was not an option.

The minutes ground by. Fran opened her e-mail and dwelled at length on each of the dozen or so items in her inbox. "Ten minutes apiece would almost get me there," she calculated. Later, she surfed the net for business news, following link after link to eat up nearly an hour. As five-thirty approached, Fran was congratulating herself when she suddenly remembered that she had never called her mother, who by now would already be making her way to the restaurant. She was committed to remaining awake for at least five more hours! While frantically searching for a way out of her predicament, it dawned on Fran that she was no longer sleepy. "How can this be," she marveled, "when I was up half the night and I haven't slept a wink all day?"

Sleep and Wakefulness Come in Waves

Fran's small revelation might have also occurred to you, yet it has only recently been given a scientific basis. It is fully possible, and actually quite common, to become more alert without first going to sleep. The traditional understanding of how one becomes sleepy (by staying awake too long) and alert (by getting some sleep) cannot readily account for this phenomenon. This age-old model was probably protected from serious challenge by its armor of common sense. Indeed, it does accurately characterize much of our experience—we do generally feel sleepy at the end of a long day and more alert if we are able to get a full night of sleep. However, it tells only half the story.

In this chapter, we complete the tale with a state-of-the-art explanation of how a robust sleep/wake cycle is formed. You will soon be immersed in a series of diagrams—perhaps dredging up anxious memories of science class. We present this material not to daunt you, but rather to give you a first glimpse of the "wave" that will carry you toward better sleep and more alert waking hours. This wave, more than sleep itself, is what you should really be seeking. To understand why, think back to those expert surfers. Sure, they require a board to pursue their sport and they have to stay fit and keep up their skills. But what surfers ultimately need is a wave—without cresting water, there is no purpose in their seeking to ride.

The same holds for sleep. You can prepare a comfortable bed, tune out the outside world, and learn to calm your inner one. All of this is important, but it is not sufficient for sleep. You must also catch a wave. To accomplish this, you will want to understand how waves of sleep and wakefulness are generated (to be reviewed shortly), how your sleeplessness is currently being maintained (revealed in the next chapter), and how to position yourself for sleep (the subject of the second part of this book). In your quest, you have a clear advantage over our exemplary surfers. They are at the mercy of the weather, the sea, and the submerged contours of the continental shelf. The best they can do is to discover the conditions that give rise to big breakers and seek these out. In contrast, you will learn how to build up your own sleep/wake cycle, to generate the very waves that will carry you off.

Simple Models of Sleep

We have discussed how the conscious mind is more effective at preventing sleep than inducing it. Fortunately, sleep is not a higher brain function. We do not have to remind ourselves to sleep or remember how to do it—even if we might sometimes think so! On some level, our bodies know how to sleep just as well as those pets whose carefree slumbers we were envying earlier. We, too, are endowed with intricate brainstem mechanisms that balance our needs for sleep and alertness.

How are these competing interests served? Given your experience with insomnia, it should not take very much reflection to see that we are not simply programmed to be alert during daylight hours and asleep at night. Regardless of our preferred bedtimes and our ability to sleep, we all spend at least some time awake and alert when it is dark outside. Sleeping during daylight hours is a bit more of a personal taste: some find it quite difficult, while others would argue that if anything, it is easier to sleep after the sun rises.

We can also safely assume that our sleep/wake cycle is not strictly dependent on our bedtimes or on the act of getting into bed. This is obvious in the case of insomnia. Wouldn't it be nice if all it took to go to sleep was to lie down? Even good sleepers following a regular bedtime schedule experience some variation with regard to when sleep actually appears. Finally, while a sleep/wake "switch," arising from the mutual inhibition of neurons promoting sleep and wakefulness, has actually been posited, we cannot place our finger directly on the toggle so as to turn sleep "on" and "off." If we could cleanly separate sleep from wakefulness, a suitable symbol for the sleep/wake cycle might be this:

Figure 1

To the contrary, you are probably painfully aware that sleep can be peppered with awakenings, and sleepiness or actual sleep can intrude into waking hours. Our state of arousal at any one moment appears to be the result of a mixture of sleepiness and alertness. We function best when one or the other clearly predominates, but we cannot always count on this to be the case. Furthermore, the states of sleep and wakefulness have some influence upon each other: the quality of our sleep is at least in part determined by how we have spent our waking hours, while our level of alertness, Fran's discovery notwithstanding, reflects to some degree how we have slept on previous nights.

Sleep clinicians and researchers have adopted the familiar yin and yang symbol to represent the sleep/wake cycle. This symbol does a better job of reflecting the interaction between sleep and wakefulness:

Figure 2

Sleepiness and Alertness Are Generated Independently

Exactly *how* sleep and wakefulness interact is a key area of inquiry for anyone contending with insomnia. In the past twenty-five years, sleep researchers have begun furnishing answers to this fundamental question. These answers are not straightforward. For starters, whether asleep or awake, we are always under the influence of *two* independent and opposing systems, which we call the Sleep Drive and the Alerting Force. This may seem counterintuitive, because the *effects* of these two systems are experienced simultaneously. Subjectively, they appear to blend, creating a single level of arousal—be that high, medium, or low. Despite this perception, the components of our state of arousal can be traced back to either the Sleep Drive or the Alerting Force, just as grains of salt and pepper retain their own characteristics when mixed in a shaker.

In your sufferings with insomnia, how many times have you reached the conclusion that your sleep is totally unpredictable? That you can feel drained of all alertness yet still be unable to sleep? That if you do manage to sleep, you will awaken for no apparent reason? That you could lie awake seemingly for nights on end without even becoming sleepy? Although other factors contribute to such maddening, haphazard experiences, the biggest obstacle to making sense of sleep and responding to insomnia effectively is a lack of appreciation for one well-documented fact: *sleepiness and alertness are generated independently*—the level of arousal we experience at any given time reflects contributions from *both* the Sleep Drive and the Alerting Force.

Being independent at their source, the two systems cannot always be counted upon to cooperate. The need for sleep, for example, can rise at the same time the force pushing us to remain alert refuses to give ground. The results of this competition can be plainly discerned in the late-evening crankiness of a wound-up five-year-old. Yet the mixing of the Sleep Drive and the Alerting Force can also yield beneficial effects, as when Fran experienced a "second wind" after a full day of battling sleep loss.

The Wave of Sleep

Figure 3 shows the sleep/wake cycle of our Ideal Sleeper. She remains alert all day. As evening approaches, her arousal level drops; she begins to feel drowsy. She gets into bed, where she quickly falls into sleep and experiences little variation in the depth of her dominant state, now sleep rather than wakefulness. As morning approaches, her arousal level rises, signaling the start of her waking day. She bounds out of bed refreshed, ready to begin the cycle anew. Commit this image to memory, for it represents the goal you are striving for—it is the perfect wave.

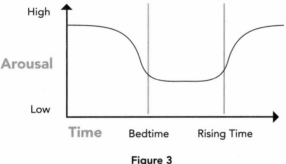

Figure 3
The ideal sleep/wake cycle

How might the Sleep Drive the Alerting Force, which we have described as independent and potentially wayward, coordinate to produce such a simple and predictable pattern? We will soon learn that while they are distinct processes, the Sleep Drive and the Alerting Force are in fact "made for each other"—their underlying properties enable a stable partnership that allows for restoration of the body and mind while also ensuring that we have sufficient dynamism to thrive in a challenging world. We will start our exploration of this complex arrangement by examining our urge to sleep.

The Sleep Drive

The course of the Sleep Drive is fairly easy to characterize. As with other physiological states that motivate behavior, such as hunger and thirst, the urge to sleep intensifies as long as we abstain from satisfying it. When we do finally sleep, the drive is gradually diminished. A simple depiction of the course of the Sleep Drive would, therefore, look something like Figure 4.

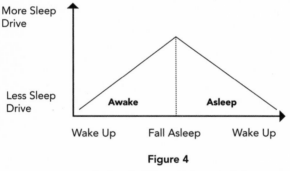

Figure 4
A simple Sleep Drive model

Notice that we are not speaking of *sleepiness* here, but rather of the underlying *Sleep Drive*. There is a big difference. To clarify this distinction, think back again to your own experience. You do not really feel progressively sleepier throughout the day, starting from the moment you awaken, even though the Sleep Drive is in fact building up relentlessly. This is because the Sleep Drive is not experienced directly. As we have discussed, the level of arousal you *do* experience (whether perceived as sleepy or alert) results from a blend of the Sleep Drive and the Alerting Force.

In actuality, the course of the Sleep Drive is slightly more complicated. It does not appear to change at the same rate indefinitely. Rather, the Sleep Drive increases at a steady rate for much of the waking day and then it begins to plateau as we approach our habitual bedtime. Once you've stayed up four hours past your bedtime, for example, the Sleep Drive is quite elevated, and it won't increase all that much if you stay up another hour or two. Conversely, much of the Sleep Drive dissipates rapidly during the first hours of sleep, but to be fully refreshed, to drain away the last vestiges of the Sleep Drive, you must accumulate a full night. A graph of its course as currently understood might look something like Figure 5.

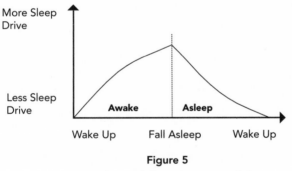

Figure 5
Real-world Sleep Drive model

Regardless of the exact shape of the segments, the key feature to remember about the Sleep Drive is this: *the Sleep Drive intensifies as we stay awake and diminishes as we sleep.*

Notice that in our model, we fall asleep when the sleep drive is very high and wake up when the drive has returned to its initial level. The effect of a night of sleep is, therefore, to return the Sleep Drive back to its starting point. Biologists term such an arrangement a *homeostatic* system because it works to maintain some function near a desirable level. The thermostat in your home works in a similar manner. It allows a certain amount of heat loss to take place before turning on your furnace. The heat of the furnace then restores your home to its initial temperature before it is automatically turned off.

While fancier home thermostats can come equipped with timers, the basic model's operation is not at all dependent upon what time it is. With a standard thermostat, how often your furnace kicks on and how long it stays on depends on nontemporal factors, such as the temperature outside and how well your home is insulated. This analogy holds for the Sleep Drive as well. It is not dependent upon time of day or night, but rather on factors such as how long you have been awake or asleep. It also depends to some extent on the nature of your waking activities and on the quality of the sleep you obtain.

A firm grasp of the workings of the Sleep Drive will prove critical as we address your insomnia. However, your understanding will be incomplete until you develop an appreciation for the dynamics of the Alerting Force, the opposing process that allows us to maintain wakefulness despite going long hours without sleep.

The Alerting Force

The rough workings of the Sleep Drive have been recognized since antiquity. By contrast, the elegant mechanisms underlying the Alerting Force have only recently been discovered, as physiologists and sleep researchers have devised ingenious experiments to tease its effects apart from those of its more straightforward counterpart. As with the Sleep Drive, the Alerting Force varies in intensity, but its fluctuations are dependent upon a clock, that is, dependent upon what time it is: *the Alerting Force has an inherent rhythm; with the passage of time, it rises and falls.*

A simple way to depict the course of the Alerting Force is presented in Figure 6.

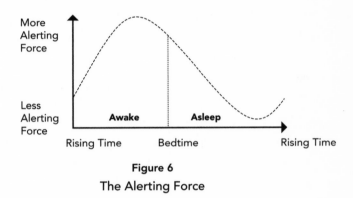

Figure 6
The Alerting Force

Notice that the valley and peak of the curve do not correspond precisely to the times when we rise from and go to sleep. When we awaken, the Alerting Force is still relatively low, but it has already begun to rise. The Alerting Force continues to gain in strength throughout the day, reaching its highest level in the evening. After it has been falling for a few hours, we typically feel ready for sleep. The Alerting Force continues to lose strength during the early and middle portions of our sleep, reaching a trough about two hours before our usual rising time. Then it begins to strengthen again and the cycle repeats.

It bears repeating that the strength of the Alerting Force is not influenced at all by how long or how well we have slept. This may be difficult to fathom, but again, a convincing example may well fall within your experience. Many of you have on occasion stayed up for an entire night by necessity. Perhaps you had to put in an emergency work shift or care for a sick child. In the first few hours after midnight, you might have had your doubts as to whether you could stay awake until morning. However, sometime around five or six o'clock, you realized that you were in the clear. We can now understand that this was because the Alerting Force was once again beginning to ascend, countering your very elevated Sleep Drive. A similar phenomenon came to the rescue of Fran at the end of her workday—in this case, the Alerting Force was ascending to its peak.

TWO MAJOR PROCESSES CONTROL YOUR SLEEP: THE SLEEP DRIVE AND THE ALERTING FORCE

The **Sleep Drive** grows stronger with each hour of wakefulness and weaker with each hour of sleep. The depth, continuity, and restorative nature of your sleep are primarily dependent upon your **Sleep Drive.**

The **Alerting Force** follows an inborn rhythm; it rises during the day to sustain alertness and falls at night to permit sleep. The **Alerting Force** is not affected by how long or how well you have slept. However, your readiness to sleep and readiness to wake up are primarily dependent upon your **Alerting Force.**

The **Alerting Force** opens a window of opportunity for sleep; the **Sleep Drive** determines how well you take advantage of that opportunity.

Circadian Rhythms

The Alerting Force rises and falls according to a biological clock. It does not follow the dictates of external clocks and wristwatches. In fact, if left to its own devices, the Alerting Force would not even follow a cycle of exactly twenty-four hours. Typically, the Alerting Force has an inherent cycle of slightly more than twenty-four hours, although occasionally it can cycle with a period of slightly less than a full day. Because its cycle length is close to that of a day, the Alerting Force is an example of a *circadian rhythm*, from the Latin *circa diēs*, meaning "about a day."

Much of our functioning as living organisms is characterized by circadian rhythmicity. A fundamental example is provided by our *core temperature* rhythm, the fluctuation of about one degree Centigrade in the temperature of our internal organs. The core body temperature rhythm is critical in terms of regulating sleep. It typically shares the same *phase*, or timing, as the Alerting Force. Indeed, the core body temperature is often measured as a proxy for the Alerting Force.

Other circadian rhythms may be out of phase with the Alerting Force but still very important for sleep. For example, the hormone *melatonin*, first secreted by the pineal gland as dusk falls, is a key factor inducing sleep. Light entering our eyes as we arise in the morning suppresses melatonin secretion, effectively telling our bodies what time it is in the outside world. *Cortisol* secretion beginning in the early morning hours is a harbinger of awakening. Good sleep depends on the synchronization of many such circadian rhythms, just as the success of a symphony depends on many musical parts appearing on cue. These internal rhythms must bear the proper *phase relationship* to each other, as well as to external rhythms such as the light/dark cycle. Finally, to pull off a restful night of sleep, this entire undulating apparatus must mesh with the homeostatic corrections of the Sleep Drive. No wonder sleeping well can seem so difficult!

We admit that the circadian physiology of sleep, even as it has been briefly alluded to and schematized here, is rather daunting. Fortunately, we can make a lot of headway toward improving your sleep by confining our discussion, going forward, to the two key concepts discussed in this chapter. With some artful blending of the Sleep Drive and the Alerting Force, we can generate big, rolling waves of sleep, identical to those traced by the Ideal Sleeper we envisioned earlier.

Building a Wave of Sleep

Despite their differing mechanisms and independent courses, we are subject to the influences of the Sleep Drive and the Alerting Force simultaneously. Our level of arousal is the result of their blending. Let's examine what happens when we look at the two functions simultaneously and then combine their effects. We will need to place the two curves on the same graph, with the same vertical axis (representing Arousal Level) and the same horizontal axis (representing Time). To accomplish this, we will have to flip one of the graphs. We choose to flip the graph of the Sleep Drive, so that values near the top of the graph will correspond to *less* Sleep Drive (and in our new series of combined graphs, More Arousal) and values near the bottom of the graph will correspond to *more* Sleep Drive (or Less Arousal). After such an adjustment, the graph of the Sleep Drive would look like this:

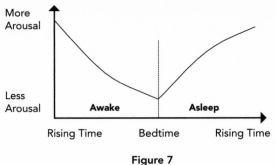

Figure 7
The Sleep Drive (flipped)

We are now ready to superimpose the two graphs:

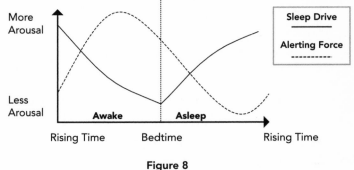

Figure 8
The Sleep Drive and the Alerting Force

Let's walk through the interactions of these two fundamental factors shaping our sleep/wake cycle, beginning from when we first rise out of bed. During much of our waking day, the increasing strength of the Alerting Force counteracts the growing strength of the Sleep Drive. (This counteraction is represented graphically by curves moving in opposite directions, as depicted by arrows in the following graph.) The result is a fairly steady level of arousal:

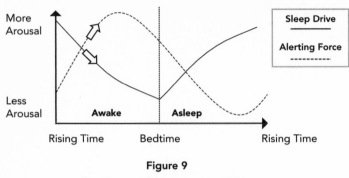

Figure 9
Daytime waking counteraction

In the evening, the two forces collude to make us sleepy—the Sleep Drive is still increasing while the Alerting Force is beginning to wane. Graphically, the two curves are both headed in the same direction, toward Less Arousal. It is this alignment that produces the steep wall of the wave that sweeps you down into sleep:

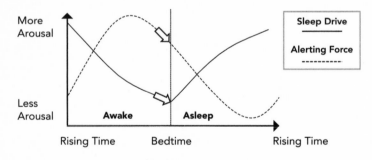

Figure 10
Evening pre-sleep alignment

During our habitual sleep period, the Sleep Drive loses strength. We are still able to keep sleeping, however, because the strength of the Alerting Force is also waning. The diminishing Sleep Drive yields More Arousal, while the diminishing Alerting Force leads to

Less Arousal. This counteraction again results in a fairly steady over-all arousal level across much of the night.

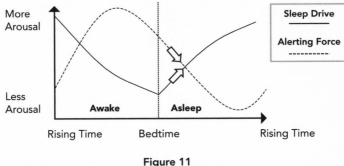

Figure 11
Nighttime sleep counteraction

Finally, about two hours before we awaken, the two forces are once more aligned. In this case, they combine to arouse us, as the Alerting Force begins to strengthen anew while the Sleep Drive continues to slowly diminish:

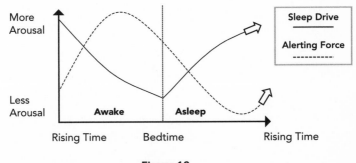

Figure 12
Morning pre-waking alignment

The alternating pattern of counteraction and alignment results in a relatively stable period of high arousal occurring through the day with a rapid decrease in arousal as bedtime approaches. A steady, low level of arousal characterizes most of the night, followed by a sharp increase in arousal in the morning. This is the pattern that characterized our hypothetical Ideal Sleeper at the beginning of this chapter:

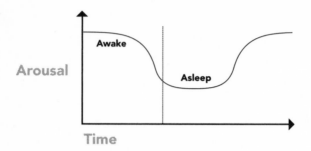

Figure 13
The sleep/wake cycle

The Sleep Drive and Alerting Force in Everyday Life

We are not ideal sleepers, and we don't adhere to ideal schedules. We might cut short our sleep on weekdays, for example, and hope to make up the difference on weekends. We may wake up in the middle of the night or nap in the middle of the day. The power of the model we have been considering is demonstrated by its ability to account for our experiences in the less-than-perfectly-regulated lives we actually live.

Suppose you miss an entire night of sleep, yet somehow drag yourself through the next day without napping. If you wait until your usual bedtime to retire, you can usually count on a long, uninterrupted sleep. This is so because your Sleep Drive has been building up in strength all the while you have been awake—it is reflecting about forty hours of continuous wakefulness rather than the sixteen or so you accumulate in a typical day. When you finally allow yourself to sleep, the Alerting Force is again on the wane and, therefore, not in a position to interfere with a deep "rebound sleep."

Now consider a related scenario, one that leads to a very different outcome, however. In this case, you have again stayed up all night, but this time you go to bed in the morning. Although you feel as if you could sleep for twelve hours, you end up awakening, groggy and irritable, after five hours or so. You did in fact build up a heightened Sleep Drive after your all-nighter, reflecting twenty-four hours of wakefulness, but now you are going to bed at the very time that the Alerting Force is picking up strength. It awakens you prematurely, preventing a full discharge of your Sleep Drive. The homeostatic mechanism that should function to maintain equilibrium has been preempted, and you must bear the consequences for the rest of the day.

If you nap in the evening, you can usually count on a harder time falling asleep later that night. The sleep you do accumulate is likely to be lighter as well. These results also follow from our discussion. Even though you are going to bed at your habitual bedtime, you have expended some of your drive for sleep prematurely, so there is less available to oppose the Alerting Force, which is still relatively strong in the first hours of the night.

Do these latter scenarios sound all too familiar? They underscore how vulnerable your sleep/wake cycle is to meddling. If you continue to respond to poor sleep with morning oversleeping, afternoon napping, watching entire movies in the middle of the night, and other maladaptive compensations, your cycle will flatten. Eventually, there will no longer be any waves for you to catch. Lest this all seem too gloomy, let us stress that a sputtering cycle may also be retuned to produce glorious waves of sleep. The choice is yours. Let's turn to an examination of these factors maintaining your insomnia (as well as those that led you to sleeplessness in the first place) so you may make an informed decision.

CHAPTER THREE

How Did I Get Insomnia?

Learning About the Three Types of Sleeplessness and How They Arise

Fogginess is a word that has often been used to describe the consequences of sleep loss, with good reason. Not only do the contours of the external world lose their sharpness, our inner experience tends to cloud over as well. Our attention wanes, limiting our exposure to new information, while old memories are less readily accessed.

With our minds so befuddled, it's hard enough to describe the general features that currently characterize our sleeplessness, let alone piece together its evolution. In this chapter, we pierce through this fog to pin down the answers to some very important questions: (1) What kind of insomnia do you have? (2) What factors brought it about? and (3) What factors are maintaining it? These are the questions that guide the clinical evaluation of patients we see in our sleep disorders centers, and they should also serve as the starting point for understanding and addressing your sleep problem.

Do You Have Insomnia?

To begin, let's consider whether you indeed have insomnia. At what point do your crummy nights add up to a formal diagnosis? Clinical criteria are available to answer this question in a relatively straightforward manner. There are three main categories of insomnia. These are difficulty falling asleep, difficulty staying asleep, and what we have called broken sleep—that is, difficulty achieving sleep that is deep, continuous, and refreshing. Clinicians also differentiate among the transient nights of sleeplessness faced by nearly everyone on occasion; acute insomnia that may set in during the weeks following a stressful event; and more entrenched, chronic cases of insomnia.

As a rule of thumb, it shouldn't take you, on average, more than thirty minutes to fall asleep. Of course, everyone has tossed and turned for an hour, or even a couple hours, now and then. Perhaps your son has taken the car out late at night for the first time. Or you sprained your back yesterday and can't get comfortable in bed. The difficulty you have falling asleep at such times is not insomnia. However, if you often take forty minutes, an hour, or longer to fall asleep—and especially if you've grown to *expect* that it will take a long time—your *difficulty falling asleep* qualifies as insomnia.

Similarly, the mere fact that you wake up during the night may not mean you have a sleep disorder. As we get older, for example, it is common to awaken for a trip to the bathroom. When you return to bed, sleep should resume within five or ten minutes. Most people will also awaken on occasion when something from their mental "to do" list rings an internal alarm. However, if you seem to have trained yourself to awaken in the middle of the night, if you are pretty much *resigned* to being unable to return to sleep and have begun instead to anticipate watching TV or surfing the web in the wee hours, your *difficulty staying asleep* amounts to insomnia as well.

Finally, we all know that some nights are better than others in terms of sleep quality. Sleep clinicians speak of the *depth* of sleep and the *continuity* of sleep as two very important characteristics determining how refreshing sleep will be. Even good sleepers may have up to a few dozen brief arousals across a night of sleep, yet these are so short—just a few seconds—that they pass unnoticed. On the other hand, if your awakenings add up to an hour or more at least three times per week, if you typically find yourself dimly aware of your surroundings and your thoughts throughout the night, if you seem to be masquerading in what passes for sleep, you have a third form of insomnia, which we call *broken sleep*.

Classifying your sleep problem in these broad terms is fairly easy. A few additional components are also required to fulfill standard criteria for insomnia. You of course need to have sufficient opportunity to sleep, under fitting circumstances. Finally, the sleep problem needs to have a negative impact on performance, mood, alertness, or other aspects of your daytime functioning. We should hasten to add that the newly revised sleep diagnostic manual used in our field, the *International Classification of Sleep Disorders-2*, takes a considerably finer-grained approach, relating insomnia to physiological disorder, psychological disturbance, distressing events, drugs or alcohol, and more. However, to get us started, the simple diagnostic scheme described here will do just fine. Answers to the other questions we posed at the outset—what brought on your insomnia and what is maintaining it—may be a bit murkier, as José's story illustrates:

At our initial interview, José sheepishly admitted how his sleepless-ness had started six years earlier. There had been no trauma, no cataclysm—just a school holiday. José hadn't made any particular plans, so with nothing else to do, he spent most of the afternoon snoozing on the sofa. After dinner he had watched a movie, still sprawled on the couch, before finally going upstairs to bed. José wasn't too surprised, therefore, when he ended up tossing and turn-ing all that night.

The next day José had struggled through a full teaching load. De-spite fortifying himself with two cups of strong coffee during after-school parent conferences, José still had felt compelled to rest for an hour or so before dinner. However, he hadn't actually fallen asleep, and after clearing the dishes, he had put in three hours grading term papers, so he was mystified and a bit alarmed when he couldn't sleep yet again that night.

José had never really considered that sleep could be a problem—at least as far as he was concerned. Sure, he had nodded sympatheti-cally as other teachers griped about being up all night. In truth, however, the notion of insomnia just didn't jibe with his experience. Previously, if he had any issue with sleep, it was how to avoid collaps-ing before bedtime! Now for the first time, José finally understood what the others were talking about. The exhaustion and craving for sleep were still present—in fact, they were stronger than ever—but somehow they couldn't push him over the edge.

It just got worse from there. José began to be distracted during his lectures. He would catch himself worrying about how much sleep he was going to get during the coming night. He bought some anti-histamines at the drugstore to promote drowsiness and later secured his first prescription sleeping pills. While the medication worked rea-sonably well, José's sleep was especially disrupted when he tried to skip nights to conserve his supply. José began to weigh his next day's obligations on an internal scale—a score of fifteen or more prompted him to reach into his stash. His weekends were now lost to napping, he had become a heavy coffee drinker, and his doctor was getting more and more reluctant to renew prescriptions. "I was a good sleeper for twenty-eight years," José bemoaned at the end of our interview. "How could it all just fall apart?"

José's story represents a fairly unusual case, in that his insomnia seemed to form out of thin air. His apprehension over the prospect of being unable to sleep, together with his changes in behavior meant to compensate for his sleeplessness (but ultimately were maladaptive in this regard), were more directly responsible for his insomnia than the innocuous trigger posed by a school holiday. At the other extreme, there certainly are instances where the source of insomnia can be traced back to a single horrific trauma. In a later chapter, we discuss the experience of Leeann, who was jarred out of a sound sleep in her own bed and raped at knifepoint. Not surprisingly, from the time of this assault onward, she was unable to sufficiently relax her state of vigilance to enter the deepest stages of sleep.

The 3P Model of Insomnia

We devised a model of insomnia some twenty years ago that has proven very useful clinically in part because it makes sense of the bewilderingly varied presentations of sleep disturbance. It helps us understand how insomnia can be the common outcome of histories as disparate as those of José and Leeann. Not only does this conception, which we now call the "3P Model of Insomnia," identify and categorize the causes of insomnia, it also points the way toward appropriate treatments for each type. It provides a rationale for treatment, motivating patients to stick with therapies even when they are initially onerous. The 3P Model is arguably the most popular framework for understanding insomnia among the community of sleep experts, and it can also help you comprehend and treat your own insomnia.

The 3P Model suggests that three distinct elements account for the onset and course of insomnia: (1) *Predisposing* **characteristics** found within individuals, that render them more susceptible to develop a particular type of insomnia; (2) *Precipitating* **events,** often outside the individual's control, that can trigger sleep disturbance, and (3) *Perpetuating* **attitudes and practices** that develop in response to the experience of insomnia and ultimately serve to maintain the sleep difficulty.

These three elements are each associated with distinct phases in the development of insomnia. **Predisposing characteristics** are operative *before* a case of insomnia actually erupts; they in fact increase the likelihood of insomnia's appearance. For example, individuals who tend to be anxious or agitated by nature require less of an external jolt to disturb their sleep. **Precipitating events** are usually readily identifiable *at the time* sleeplessness becomes acute. Indeed, they are often explicitly tagged as "the cause" of the problem. For example, a new mother might complain, "I was a great sleeper until my daughter was born—now she gets through the night just fine, but I still can't sleep." **Perpetuating attitudes and practices** come into play *after* insomnia has made its appearance, as the poor sleeper struggles to cope with the problem. They are often responsible for

the transformation of a period of acute sleeplessness into chronic insomnia, as we saw in José's case.

Perpetuating attitudes and practices usually present the best opportunity to bring about quick improvement in sleep quality. After
all, predisposing characteristics by nature are likely to be deep
seated, and precipitating events may be either in full bloom (and,
therefore, exceedingly difficult to contain) or already buried in the
past. Let's examine each of these components of the 3P Model in
closer detail.

PREDISPOSING CHARACTERISTICS

As introduced earlier, individual traits or characteristics may set the
stage for insomnia. Many such factors appear to be present on an *inherited* basis—indeed, these are likely to be responsible for the quick
emergence in infancy of the "good sleepers" and "poor sleepers" we
discussed earlier. But sometimes, it's an *acquired* characteristic that
indirectly leads to insomnia. For example, an old shoulder injury
may have left you some residual discomfort that is not sufficiently
intense in itself to lead to sleeplessness. However, by lurking in the
background, this pain lowers your threshold for insomnia. It may
take less noise outside your window at two A.M. or a smaller problem
to be faced tomorrow to upset your sleep than would otherwise be
the case. Whether inherited or acquired, predisposing factors are
typically overlooked even when they are in plain sight, precisely because they predate the onset of the disorder. Let's take a closer look
at some inherited characteristics that may predispose to insomnia, so
that if you recognize them in yourself you can take preventative
measures to preserve your sleep.

Physiological Hyperarousal

Some people seem to operate in a higher gear, regardless of the particular circumstances they find themselves in. They were literally born that way. These individuals are said to exhibit *hyperarousal*, which can be reflected in such physiological measures as an increased heart rate, heightened muscle tension, faster brain waves, a higher metabolic rate, and elevated hormone levels. The mechanism known as the hypothalamic-pituitary-adrenal (HPA) axis, which responds to stress with cortisol secretion and readiness for "fight or flight," has been hypothesized to predispose individuals toward insomnia. Heightened cortisol levels may linger even when the stressor is no longer present.

Hyperaroused individuals often report that they have had lifelong sleep problems and that their sleep only goes from bad to worse when stressed. The issues they point to as the cause of their sleeplessness may strike others as relatively minor. Even following protracted sleep loss, their recovery sleep is not particularly deep and satisfying. We can infer that their HPA axis is easily and frequently triggered, producing chronic hyperarousal.

Perhaps you count yourself among this hyperaroused group. On good days, you feel lucky to be so constituted. You feel more responsive than the usual plodder—more attuned to the world, more vital. On bad days, however, these same juiced-up reactions compel you toward restlessness, jumpiness, and irritability. What may come as a surprise to you is that insofar as sleep is concerned, both manifestations of hyperarousal—the positive as well as the negative—are harmful. Sleep prefers neutrality, a state not often experienced by those predisposed to physiological hyperarousal.

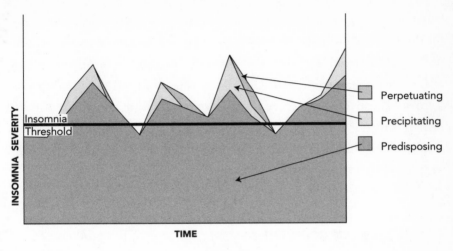

Figure 14
Predisposing Characteristics Contributing to Insomnia Over Time

While Figure 14 depicts all three factors in the 3P Model at work, it illustrates how Predisposing characteristics may be primary in a given case, and how people who possess strong risk factors for insomnia, such as physiological hyperarousal, may be prone to episodic insomnia. Arousal is easy to trigger in these individuals, whereas dampening this activation after stress hormones have flooded their systems or excitatory impulses have stampeded through their brains may be harder to achieve. Figure 14 illustrates a Predisposing characteristics so strong that it takes only very small precipitating events to induce repeated bouts of sleeplessness.

Cognitive Hyperarousal

Hyperarousal can also be cognitive in nature. Some individuals' minds are rarely at rest, unable to sustain a contemplative mental state. Do you recognize yourself as someone who is given over to obsessive worrying, to second-guessing, or to racing thoughts? Do you internalize your conflicts, mentally airing various viewpoints so relentlessly that your mind begins to resemble a cable news channel? All of this cognitive activation not only inhibits sleep onset, it can also alter the experience of what sleep you finally manage to obtain. Typically, you may perceive your sleep to be lighter than it should be. In more extreme cases, you may perceive yourself as being awake, even during periods that would be scored on a polysomnograph as moderately deep sleep.

INDICATORS OF COGNITIVE AND PHYSIOLOGICAL HYPERAROUSAL

- Mind racing
- Constant worrying
- Rapid speech
- Muscle tension
- Agitation and restlessness
- Tension headaches
- Heart pounding
- Feeling unable to take a deep breath
- Cold hands and feet
- Inability to nap
- "Hairtrigger" startle response
- Anxiety

"Night Owls" and "Morning Larks"

Most people can readily identify themselves as morning or evening types. "Morning larks" are "early to bed, early to rise." They enjoy awakening to the sensation of warm yellow sunlight streaming across their faces early on summer mornings. They have a hearty appetite for breakfast and a lot of energy to tackle work assignments at the beginning of the day. That energy falls off precipitously later in the evening, so it takes a special effort to attend late-night social engagements.

By contrast, "night owls" don't come into their own until the sun goes down. They abhor morning light. They sleep with bedroom curtains drawn tight, as late into the morning or afternoon as their obligations allow. They are likely to skip breakfast but may add a second dinner late at night before retiring to bed. If night owl types must work a regular nine-to-five job, they drag themselves through most of the day and just begin to feel fully awake by the end of their shift. Owls tend to gravitate toward night work or occupations with flexible hours. For example, they are easy to spot among musicians, computer programmers, and ER nurses.

Circadian "morningness" vs. "eveningness," as these tendencies are also known, are included in our model as Predisposing characteristics because there is evidence that, in their extreme forms, they have a genetic basis. For morning larks working day jobs, the low point of their circadian temperature rhythm (a marker for the Alerting Force) occurs slightly more than two hours before their typical weekday rising time, perhaps around four or five in the morning. Night owls tend to have a delayed temperature rhythm. Their cycle may not bottom out until perhaps eight or nine A.M. so they can easily sleep to ten or eleven A.M. if given the chance. The peaks of their temperature rhythm will also be correspondingly delayed, which is one reason why night owls feel so energized late at night. Figure 15 returns to what should be a familiar depiction of the Alerting Force to illustrate phase differences between morning larks and night owls.

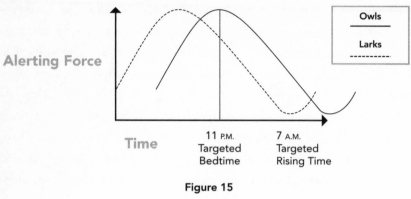

Alerting Force

Owls

Larks

- - - - - - - - - -

Time

11 P.M.
Targeted
Bedtime

7 A.M.
Targeted
Rising Time

Figure 15
Larks and owls

The figure shows that at eleven P.M., a typical target bedtime for high school students on a school night or for day-shift workers, the core temperature rhythm is well past its peak for morning larks. It is relatively easy for them to fall asleep on this falling portion of their temperature cycle, and soon temperatures will be quite low, helping to maintain sleep through the night. For night owls, by contrast, the temperature rhythm may be just peaking at eleven P.M. Sleep will be the last thing on their minds at this hour. A similar divergence occurs on the morning side. For larks, the temperature cycle is already rising at seven A.M., mobilizing them out of bed, whereas the cycle has not yet even bottomed out for owls, prompting them to bury their heads under the blankets and keep sleeping.

Earlier, we stated that the difference between morning and evening types appears to be a stable, inherited trait. What is actually inherited is not the specific timing of the temperature cycle or other circadian rhythms. The peaks and troughs of these cycles are not fixed. They are in fact quite susceptible to change by light exposure, physical activity, social stimulation, and other factors. Whenever we cross time zones by jet plane, the resulting "jet lag" corresponds in large measure to the discrepancy between our circadian rhythms (initially still regulated according to our home time zone) and the time cues of our new environment—but this discrepancy dwindles as our internal circadian cycles shift to align with the new time zone.

What we *do* inherit is the biological clock that imparts rhythmicity to all our physiological functions. We have learned that this clock has an inherent period of about twenty-four hours—usually just a few minutes longer. If we were to be isolated from all time cues, this *"free-running"* period length would be expressed in our temperature cycle and other rhythms. The peak of our daily temperature rhythm, for example, might arrive a few minutes later on Monday than on Sunday, and yet a few more minutes later on Tuesday. Normally, we make up this slight discrepancy by "resetting" our internal clocks on a daily basis, just as we might continually adjust a faulty but still prized heirloom clock on our nightstand.

However, it is harder for some people to make this internal adjustment. The pressure for peaks and troughs to drift later can be so strong in these individuals that free running may occur even when time cues are available but not particularly salient. For example, some teenagers on a summer break may go to bed and rise progressively later for several nights in a row—each of their "days" on this kind of free-running schedule is actually longer than twenty-four hours. Researchers have discovered that when people with such slow-running clocks do "entrain" to a regular twenty-four-hour day (say, when September rolls around and they have to begin attending classes), they tend to have later temperature peaks as well as other phase delays. They are the night owl types we have been discussing. In severe cases, circadian phase delay can lead to significant psychosocial distress (e.g., suspension from school or the workplace due to persistent tardiness), and clinicians may diagnose a specific sleep disorder known as *Delayed Sleep Phase Disorder*.

If you are a night owl, your bedtime may be later than usual, but under normal circumstances, you can still fall asleep reasonably quickly and garner enough sleep to wake up without too much difficulty. Under stressful conditions, however, you will have more trouble winding down and falling asleep. You will require extra time to "decompress" and ready yourself for sleep. Conversely, if you are a morning lark, your tendency will be to respond to stress with an early morning awakening, because your underlying circadian rhythms are already tugging you toward wakefulness at an earlier hour.

Anxiety and Depression

It will hardly come as a surprise that psychological distress leads to problems sleeping. Both anxiety and depression bring psychophysiological changes that interfere with sleep onset and sleep maintenance. Good sleep is nurtured in a bed of ease, a sense of composure with regard to the past, the present, and the future. It requires assurance that the challenges of the day have been handled appropriately, and at least temporary absolution for sins remembered from years past. The ability to sleep also depends on our feeling secure, allowing us to temporarily drop our guard for seven or so hours, against both desperadoes breaking through windows and distressing thoughts breaking through into consciousness. Ultimately, some degree of confidence and hopefulness about the future is also a prerequisite for restful sleep. If we are convinced that the coming day will be even just manageable (let alone wonderful), we will take the shortcut to tomorrow that sleep provides. Otherwise, we will stay where we are, rooted in the present, and make wary preparations for dealing with the future all night long.

Anxiety recruits many of the same "fight or flight" reactions we have been considering under the heading of hyperarousal. It can inhibit sleep outright through heart racing, muscle tightening, obsessive thinking, or other means. Alternatively, anxiety may allow us to succumb to the first hours of sleep, when the drive for deep NREM sleep is greatest, only to lead to awakenings when that drive has been partially sated. We all have a few dozen very brief arousals, even during good nights of sleep. Anxious thoughts may lie in wait, in some recess of our sleeping mind, and poke through one of these arousals when they get the chance, stretching what should have been just a few seconds of relatively fast electroencephalographic (EEG) waves into a full-blown awakening lasting minutes or hours.

Depression is associated with disruptive changes in sleep architecture. People who are depressed spend more time awake at night, whether at the beginning, middle, or end. They accumulate less of the deepest NREM sleep stages, while a greater proportion of total sleep time may be devoted to REM sleep, often accompanied by vivid, disturbing dreams.

Depression is also characterized by alterations of biological rhythms. Early morning awakenings are a hallmark of Major Depressive Disorder. Sleep duration may be shortened to four or five hours. There may also be a phase advance of REM sleep, leading to a shortened interval between the time of falling asleep and the first appearance of REM sleep. Instead of the typical eighty or ninety minutes, this REM latency may be just forty or fifty minutes. In general, the nightly allotment of REM sleep is concentrated more toward the earlier sleep cycles.

In addition to its direct effects on sleep, depression changes the nature of our waking behavior. We become lethargic and withdrawn, more prone to stay indoors and less likely to reach peaks of physical activation and social engagement. Given the interdependence of sleep and wakefulness, this in turn interferes with subsequent sleep. The end result of such a downward spiral is illustrated by a patient of ours named David:

David had a hard time filling up a free hour with anything of interest. The notion of pursuing a hobby or recreational activity seemed utterly foreign. He stared blankly at neighbors tending their gardens, at his old classmates still joining softball leagues. What was the point? David functioned best when he managed to have overlapping obligations that could pull him from one moment to the next. Left on his own, he was at a loss, lying on the couch or twisted up in his stale sheets.

David's hopelessness was most acute during the nighttime, when it seemed to him that everyone else was with a partner, capping off their days with sex and sleep. It was too much to deal with in a darkened bedroom. So David stayed in the living room with the lights on. He didn't have the patience to read. While the television blared nonstop, he hardly heard it anymore. Sleep came in one- or two-hour packets, usually sometime in the evening, again around two in the morning, and occasionally around six-thirty, just before he had to drag himself off the couch for work.

When sleep has so thoroughly dissipated amidst the bleakness of depression, not much improvement may be expected until the mood disorder itself has been addressed.

PRECIPITATING EVENTS

When we find ourselves suddenly unable to sleep, it's natural to ask ourselves why. Most of the time we can come up with an answer, and when we do, it generally involves what is called a Precipitating event in our 3P Model of Insomnia. Precipitating events are usually easy to spot. They are changes in routine that throw both our waking lives and our sleep out of balance. Precipitating events often arrive abruptly, as with the pain triggered by a herniated disc, the grief of losing a loved one, the disorientation of retirement, or the anxiety touched off by assuming new work responsibilities. Precipitating events can also build gradually, such as when tensions mount in a failing marriage or when a student falls behind on a semester's coursework.

Occasionally, Precipitating events are not so easily identified. This may be because their contribution toward sleeplessness is actually insignificant when compared to the role played by Predisposing characteristics or Perpetuating attitudes and practices. This was the case for José, whom we met at the start of this chapter. In other instances, Precipitating events may in fact be important but still overlooked because they appear to be so innocuous. Such was the case with another patient we treated named Sherry:

Sherry had been a good sleeper for all of her thirty-four years. She couldn't then understand why, with her marriage off to a great start, good health, and a career that was growing ever more successful, she would now be experiencing difficulty falling asleep. Sure, things were changing in her life, but these changes were all for the better.

Upon taking a careful history, it turned out that Sherry had adjusted her bedtime nearly an hour earlier to match her husband's schedule, which was dictated by his need for more sleep and his earlier starting time at work. Although she wasn't particularly sleepy at this earlier hour, Sherry wanted to start each night together. Because her bedtimes had often varied an hour or so from night to night before her marriage, Sherry hadn't thought that the change would be consequential.

This shift of bedtime was in fact the key Precipitating event for Sherry's insomnia. The combination of trying to advance the timing of her sleep phase (always a risky proposition for sleep compared to delaying bedtime, given the built-in lag of our biological clocks) and consistently accumulating more time in bed (because she was still rising at the same morning hour) had set her up for difficulty initiating sleep.

At first, Sherry tried getting up earlier as well, to keep the amount of time she spent in bed constant. However, this earlier schedule ultimately disagreed with her "night-owl" tendencies. Instead, she grew comfortable climbing into bed with her husband to snuggle for a while, later to slip out to an easy chair and spend some quiet moments catching up on her reading. This adjustment allowed Sherry time to wind down and ready herself for sleep.

PERPETUATING ATTITUDES AND PRACTICES

When most people suffer through a poor night of sleep, they feel sleepy the next day. This response may seem too trivial to merit comment, yet it represents perhaps our main defense against chronic insomnia. Sleep is supposed to be self-correcting: sleep loss increases the drive for sleep; it incurs a "sleep debt." This debt should be experienced as increased sleepiness during waking hours. It should then lead to more sleep of deeper intensity when bedtime rolls around again, which in turn should pay back the sleep debt.

So how can such a simple feedback mechanism fail? Why is it that one poor night of sleep is so often followed by another? The problem may have less to do with your sleep and more with the way you cope with sleeplessness. Each disastrous night may trigger shifts in your thoughts and attitudes about sleep, your confidence, your behaviors surrounding bedtime, your diet, sleep schedule, and other key determinants of sleep quality. You may think these changes are compensating for loss of sleep, but in fact they often serve to prolong the sleep problem. That is why we call them Perpetuating attitudes and practices in our 3P Model.

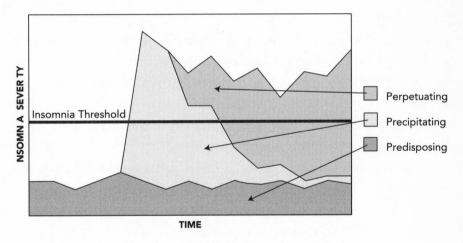

Figure 16
A stressful event precipitates insomnia. The stress resolves but sleeplessness persists, perpetuated by maladaptive attitudes and practices.

Extending Bedtime to Gain More Sleep

One of the most common Perpetuating practices maintaining insomnia is spending too much time in bed, whether actually catching up on sleep or merely trying to sleep. This tactic is certainly understandable, given the toll of fatigue, sleepiness, mood disturbance, and diminished ability to think clearly that sleep loss exacts. If these symptoms can be reversed by catching up on sleep, why not retire to bed early, sleep late in the morning, and stay in bed for hours on end, even when you are unable to sleep? After all, it stands to reason that the more time you spend in bed, the more sleep you are likely to get.

The main problem with this coping strategy is one it shares with virtually all the other Perpetuating factors we will consider: it may help in the short run, but its long-term consequences are harmful. Sure, on some occasions you will in fact get more sleep if you climb into bed early. However, on other occasions, this practice will lead to a short stint of sleep followed by prolonged middle-of-the-night awakenings, with sleep finally returning in the morning hours. Spending extra time in bed will generally increase night-to-night variability, so you will never know what kind of sleep you'll be getting on a given night. This in turn will stoke anticipatory anxiety about the whole endeavor of getting to sleep.

Oversleeping in the morning to make up for sleep loss brings an additional peril. Although it may provide immediate relief, it will also cause you to miss out on time cues such as early morning light exposure that help generate a consistent sleep cycle. Your sleep rhythm will tend to drift later, leading to more difficulty falling asleep on subsequent nights and increased anxiety regarding bedtime, perpetuating a vicious cycle.

Using Naps and Stimulants to Counter Sleep Loss

Daytime napping may indeed perk you up, but at the cost of diminishing your Sleep Drive. We're sure you've met many people who swear by their daytime naps, and indeed in some cultures, naps can be considered a norm, as exemplified by the siesta. However, a prolonged mid-day nap is generally paired with a later bedtime and a shorter nocturnal sleep period to create a sustainable pattern. It's when you try to have it both ways—getting in a full complement of sleep at night as well as a daytime nap—that you are likely to run into trouble.

Less often appreciated is that a brief nod in the evening, or even just hovering at the edge of sleep while watching TV, may make it difficult to fall asleep later that night. Guiding yourself into sleep is similar to the challenge facing a pilot approaching a runway: you have to gauge your distance from bedtime and adjust your "altitude" accordingly. If you glide down too close to sleep early in the evening and then have to "pull up" into wakefulness to get ready for bed, you will no longer be ready for sleep. Just as a student pilot will have to circle the airfield and try again, you may have to wait a while for the next wave of sleepiness and another opportunity to ease yourself into sleep.

It can seem at times that caffeine is the core fuel of our society. Once obtained primarily and unceremoniously with our morning cup of coffee or in a carbonated soda beverage, caffeine has infiltrated nearly every hour and venue of our waking life. Wherever we find ourselves, caffeine is close at hand, warmed enticingly in glass or stainless containers. It is served up within frothy concoctions on nearly every street corner, blended into over-the-counter preparations, and packed into energizing "pick-me-ups" lining convenience store shelves. Whereas nicotine, its erstwhile partner, has of late been relegated to furtive positions out on the sidewalk or the backyard, caffeine can still be enjoyed everywhere.

While the divergent fates of caffeine and nicotine can certainly be justified on the basis of their potential for harm, caffeine is hardly benign. When it comes to compensating for sleep loss, caffeine is a mixed blessing. On the positive side, its stimulant properties clearly make you more alert and able to function, despite sleep loss. However, it will also interfere with subsequent sleep. Caffeine is a potent, long-acting stimulant, with a half life typically ranging between three and seven hours (although it can be much longer in the aged, in individuals who have liver problems, in those who are pregnant or taking oral contraceptives, or in those who are using other medications that interfere with its metabolism). What this means in practice is that the double cappuccino you linger over after work, which contains upward of 200 milligrams caffeine, is still egging you on at midnight. Its residual effect, as you are trying to fall asleep, is roughly equivalent to what would be expected from drinking a cup of regular coffee just before bedtime. When you do finally manage to sleep, your EEG patterns will show discernable effects from that single hefty dose all the way to the end of the night—even though it was consumed more than twelve hours earlier!

Insomniacs who rely too heavily on caffeine to compensate for poor sleep often develop a condition known as *caffeinism*, characterized by restlessness, anxiety, cardiac arrhythmia, gastrointestinal distress, irritability, and other complaints. While tolerance to these effects of caffeine may develop in habitual users, other problems such as headaches, drowsiness, and lethargy can appear with a vengeance when attempts are made to withdraw from the substance. A surprising number of our patients defend their decision to rely on caffeine, even after their problems have prompted the effort and expense of visiting a sleep specialist. We often hear the claim, "I can drink coffee some nights and go straight to sleep—it doesn't have any effect on me." Far from indicating a benign condition, such a boast suggests that caffeine intake may be especially problematic. It may indicate that tolerance has developed to the immediate alerting effect of caffeine, allowing sleep onset to occur, while subsequent sleep quality remains impaired. It might also suggest that a considerable sleep debt has accrued, to the extent that the stimulating effect of caffeine is overridden.

In recent years, we have encountered a new variation on this theme of using a stimulant to compensate for insomnia. Modafinil, a nonamphetamine stimulant originally developed to treat the excessive daytime sleepiness present in patients suffering from narcolepsy, has gained a wider following. At first, physicians started using the drug to treat fatigue present in other neurological disorders, such as Multiple Sclerosis. Then the medication began to turn up in shift workers or those following an irregular sleep/wake schedule (such as truckers), who used it to make up for the inevitable sleep loss these schedules entail. Now we are occasionally seeing the drug used to treat the daytime consequences of insomnia. It might be argued that when compared with the cost and sleep-disruptive effects of the double cappuccino discussed earlier, modafinil represents a reasonable alternative. Our concern here, amplified in the next section, is with making a habit of ceding control over our state of consciousness to any external agent.

When we stress the harmful effects of Perpetuating attitudes and practices to people with long-standing histories of insomnia, we are sometimes met with incredulity. Such patients concede that these mechanisms might be operative for others, but they just do not jibe with personal experience. They insist that their sleep is random, impervious to manipulation, whether for good or ill. They can recall sleeping wonderfully after ingesting large amounts of both caffeine and alcohol. At other times, they have sworn off these substances, and naps to boot, only to experience one of their worst weeks of sleep ever.

In fact, reduced responsiveness to factors that normal sleepers would find disruptive or sleep-enhancing may characterize a subgroup of very poor sleepers. Their sleep/wake cycles have become attenuated after years of compensating for chronically disturbed sleep, to the point where they do not perceive much difference between day and night. Their sleep is broken and light, and their wakefulness is drowsy and lacking in vigor. Under these conditions, a double cappuccino may not suffice to keep alertness buoyed, nor would abstaining from it assure a better night's sleep. The caffeine's effect would be akin to that of a pebble thrown into a choppy lake—essentially lost amidst the chaos. If this scenario applies to you, it is important to recognize that your insensitivity is more a reflection of the sorry state of your sleep than evidence that you can disregard Perpetuating factors with impunity.

Sleep Aids

In our thirty years of clinical practice, we have encountered relatively few chronic insomniacs who have not resorted at one time or another to sleeping pills in the hopes of improving their sleep. Indeed, many patients come to us with the goal, endorsed if not set by their physicians, of getting off drugs. (People who make the effort to find a sleep specialist are, of course, not representative of the entire population of poor sleepers. Most people contending with chronic insomnia do not use sleeping pills, and some sleep experts question whether *hypnotic* medications—the technical name for sleeping pills—are in fact underutilized, especially when compared with poor alternatives such as over-the-counter sedating preparations or alcohol.)

In earlier generations, the perils associated with barbiturate overdose appeared to have cast a stigma over the use of sleeping pills. The development of benzodiazepines such as Halcion and Dalmane, with their improved ratios of benefits to risks, brought about greater acceptance of the use of drugs formulated specifically to treat sleep disturbance, although they, too, generated public mistrust amidst reports of memory loss, morning hangover, agitation, and other problems. Newer nonbenzodiazepine agents such as Ambien and Sonata are both quite effective in promoting sleep and more selective in their actions. Currently, we are experiencing a sea change in the recommended use and marketing of some sleeping pills, as they are shedding their traditional status as agents for the temporary relief of sleep disturbance (medicines to be used for up to a few weeks in times of acute stress to "get back on track") to allow for potentially longer-term administration.

Although at the time of writing only one compound has completed the clinical trials necessary to establish effectiveness over the long term, out in the real world, patients have been conducting their own impromptu "trials" for years. Anecdotal evidence suggests that responses to long-term use of sleeping pills are quite variable. Some individuals have indeed been taking the same standard dose nightly for years and accumulate six to eight hours of satisfying sleep using this method. (You may be wondering why these satisfied sleepers show up at the offices of sleep specialists! Oftentimes, it's a matter of impatience on the part of prescribing physicians that prompts their visits, rather than any subjective complaints.)

Long-term sleeping pill use can be less than completely satisfying in a number of ways. Some poor sleepers complain that the best they can do with their pills is four or five hours of sleep that somehow is perceived as "drugged," but they continue to use the medications because their sleep is worse without them. Others can count at most on one or two good nights when using sleeping pills, followed by a loss of effectiveness. These patients often pick and choose their nights of drug administration, depending upon how exhausted they are, what obligations they face the next day, and the extent of their remaining drug supply. Finally, there are those whose agitated minds and bodies are easily able to override a standard hypnotic dose. They end up routinely doubling the dosage at bedtime, perhaps to be supplemented by yet another pill or fraction thereof if an awakening becomes too prolonged in the middle of the night. This group typically finds it difficult to maintain a supply of medication from a single physician and engages in the various drug-seeking ploys characteristic of classic substance abusers. In our experience, it is the relatively rare insomniac who reaches this point. The vast majority of those taking sleeping pills are able to responsibly manage their use, albeit with varying levels of satisfaction.

Reliance on sleeping medications is a Perpetuating practice in our 3P Model, in part because of their pharmacological effects. They usually lead to sleep of middling quality—not fully satisfying but good enough to put off seeking other solutions. They also lead to some degree of agitation and arousal if the patient stops taking them abruptly, known in the context of sleep disorders as "rebound insomnia." While this withdrawal syndrome may be relatively muted for the newer hypnotic agents, with symptoms that vary in intensity across individuals, it is often present in sufficient degree to contribute at least in part toward chronic drug use.

The main reason sleeping pill usage qualifies as a Perpetuating factor for insomnia, however, has more to do with psychology than pharmacology. The psychological literature contains a concept known as the "locus of control" that is quite relevant to this discussion. Each of us has a "locus of control"—the subjective perception that our actions are motivated primarily through internally generated efforts or via externally imposed forces. For example, a classroom of students may all read the same "rags-to-riches" story. Some students, oriented toward an "internal locus of control," might attribute the heroine's rise primarily to her perseverance, kindness, or ingenuity, whereas others with an "external locus of control" might suggest that she happened to be in the right place at the right time, or that she benefited from others going out of their way to help an attractive young woman.

People who use sleeping pills regularly tend to attribute their ability to sleep to the pill itself. They have an external locus of control with regard to sleep. This is so even though the use of a sleeping pill is actually a collaborative effort. (After all, sleeping pills are not a form of general anesthesia, knocking out a completely passive patient. The would-be sleeper has to achieve some degree of repose in bed for the pill to work effectively.) By attributing the appearance of decent sleep wholly to their medication, chronic users of sleeping pills feel at a loss when they attempt to sleep on their own. Lacking access to the source of sleep, they can only expect a poor night. Growing tense and frustrated in their beds, this prophecy is soon enough fulfilled, reinforcing the notion that the return to sleep will indeed require a return to medication.

We recognize that there are advantages to hypnotic medications that may render them appropriate in some cases, which will be specified in later chapters. They produce a rapid response—usually on the first night—and they require less effort on the part of the poor sleeper to see improvement than other therapies. Therefore, although our program is primarily intended to improve your sleep through cognitive/behavioral treatment, we will make some general comments on medication strategies.

If you mainly have trouble falling asleep, you should be taking your medication so it is effective when you turn out the lights. Most hypnotics reach their maximum effectiveness about one hour after administration. Therefore, taking a pill about forty-five minutes prior to lights out makes sense. If you start to get too sleepy before bedtime, you should reduce the dose or take it closer to lights out. Medication with a short *half life*—the time it takes for the amount of drug in the body to be reduced by one-half—would be the rational choice for difficulty falling asleep.

If you primarily have trouble staying asleep, your strategy should be quite different. To maximally extend your sleep with a hypnotic, you should take the drug just before you turn off the lights. Use of a medication with a longer half life is likely to be more effective in helping you stay asleep, or helping you fall back to sleep more easily if you do wake up.

With the development of hypnotics having very short half lives, a new strategy of dosing in the middle of the night has emerged. If you have no trouble falling asleep but experience fragmented sleep starting in the middle of the night, taking a medication with a very short half life at your first awakening will specifically target the second half of your sleep. A cautionary note needs to be sounded—drug hangover in the morning may still result for some, bringing irksome sleepiness and memory problems or even dangerous falls.

Some people are able to calmly decide on which nights to use sleeping pills, based on the level of stress they are experiencing, while others get caught up in obsessive night-by-night decision-making. Our suggestion is that if medication is indicated, for example in the midst of a crisis, simply take it as prescribed. Similarly, when coming off sleeping pills, work with your doctor to devise a tapering schedule, and stick to it. Many patients constantly experiment with what pill to take, how much to take, and when to take it. Such indecision betrays lack of confidence in their chosen therapy. Some sleeplessness is to be expected during the active treatment of insomnia, whether or not medication is being employed. Occasional nights of disturbed sleep do not call for changing therapeutic course.

Counterproductive Beliefs and Attitudes About Sleep

The final set of factors perpetuating insomnia we will consider are alterations in beliefs and attitudes about sleep that in turn affect sleep itself. As we have discussed, people who do not sleep well end up doing a lot more thinking about sleep and about themselves as sleepers—and much of this extra thinking is decidedly unhelpful. Chiefly, poor sleepers experience an alteration in their self-image. As a fundamental aspect of life veers out of control and their daytime functioning plummets, insomniacs develop a general sense of vulnerability. Their self-esteem, sense of well-being, and mood are all threatened. Their quality of life suffers, leading to an ever greater focus on sleep. The vicious cycle of worrying about sleeplessness leading to increased arousal leading to worsening sleep is an all too common outcome.

In addition to changes in self-image, the experience of insomnia leads to distortions in attitudes and beliefs about sleep itself. For example, you may be under the misconception that everyone needs eight hours of sleep to function. If you average only six to seven hours nightly, you might come to believe that the ensuing sleep debt will lead to a wide array of problems, including premature aging, immune system compromise, and a total inability to function at work. A feeling of catastrophe is set in motion, a conviction that insomnia is ruining your life. Again, such a heightened state of alert is anything but conducive to sleep. It is also based on a distorted reading of the scientific literature. While it is becoming increasingly evident that sleep is tied to our well-being on many levels, it is also true that there is widespread variability in how much sleep individuals need and a considerable amount of resiliency and adaptability built into the sleep-wake system.

We do not wish to downplay the fact that sleep deprivation is a serious problem, both for individuals and for society as a whole. Whether people who cut short their time in bed are choosing to do so voluntarily or responding to circumstances beyond their control, they can expect to experience troublesome sleepiness and perhaps inadvertent dozing or regular napping as well. Sleepiness is also associated with performance deficits; it is one of the major causes of fatal motor vehicle accidents and has been a key factor underlying many industrial and commercial transportation calamities. We are gratified that the media are finally waking up to the dangers sleepiness poses. Why then are we not more strident in our warnings to you about these perils, given that so many of you are losing sleep?

First, sleep deprivation is different from insomnia. In contrast to the consistently short sleep sandwiched between work shifts by the moonlighter trying to make ends meet, sleep duration is typically quite variable in people with insomnia. There are the horrendous nights, yes, but these are interspersed between others that are just mediocre and perhaps a few when complete collapse is followed by some recovery sleep. While a particularly poor night's sleep may indeed result in bleary-eyed somnolence, in general, fatigue, lack of energy, and irritability are more common consequences of insomnia than sleepiness. Studies have shown that unlike sleep-deprived individuals, insomniacs actually have difficulty falling asleep during the day when given the opportunity.

Second, cataloguing the harmful consequences of sleep loss would more likely lead to anxiety and roadblocks than spur helpful changes in your attitudes and behavior. Given that you are reading this book, we expect that you are already motivated to work to resolve your problem. We will, therefore, stay focused on fostering the understanding and self-assurance you need to get to sleep.

You will sleep best if you understand the **three targets** for insomnia treatment.

Predisposing characteristics render you more susceptible to developing a particular type of insomnia:

- Cognitive hyperarousal
- Physiological hyperarousal
- Emotional reactivity
- Your "feel-best rhythm" (evening vs. morning)

Precipitating events, often outside your control, can trigger sleep disturbance:

- Family conflicts
- Work-related stress
- Health issues
- Death of a loved one or other loss

Perpetuating attitudes and practices develop in response to sleeplessness but ultimately serve to maintain insomnia:

- Getting into bed early
- Staying in bed late
- Spending extra time in bed
- Napping
- Caffeine
- Sleep medications
- Worrying about sleep or daytime functioning

• • •

At this point, you possess a basic background on the subject of insomnia, distilled both from current research and best clinical practices, to go along with the intimate firsthand familiarity with the disorder you have gained through hard experience. You have come to comprehend why sleep can be so unreliable and how both your mind and body stand ready to sacrifice sleep, at least for the moment, if necessary to achieve greater security. You appreciate the role played by socialization, how parental expectations regarding sleep are internalized by the child, leading to performance anxiety. You have a fledgling understanding of the interactive nature of the Sleep Drive and the Alerting Force, of how they can combine to create a wave of sleep or merely get in each other's way. You have learned how different factors predispose some people to insomnia, precipitate the disturbance, and perpetuate its misery.

We will soon be pulling all this knowledge together to work for you. Not to "take control of your sleep"—hopefully even the most cursory reader will have understood by now that we would consider such a rallying cry to be foolhardy and ill-fated. Rather, we will help you align yourself with sleep, to make your peace with its tidal pull, and let yourself be carried off. In the second half of this book, we will be recommending all kinds of changes to the ways you spend your days, evenings, and nights. We will reconsider your evening activities, your bedtime rituals, the time you get into bed and how long you stay there, and what you do when you are unable to sleep. Before all this behavior modification gets under way, however, we have one last bit of prep work to do. We need to get you thinking about what sleep *means* to you.

CHAPTER FOUR

What Does Sleep Mean to Me?

Challenging Your Beliefs About Sleep

As a rule, things do not occur merely because we think about them. We can imagine ourselves winning the lottery all day long; the odds are still about ten million to one against it happening. Mental visualization might help us improve our bowling approach or golf swing, but we still need to enlist our muscles to move the ball. Willing something into being is generally beyond the abilities of mere mortals. Hypochondriacs might count themselves lucky that this is so. Their preoccupation with illness, troubling as it may be, fortunately does not suffice to bring on disease.

Insomnia is an exception to this rule, because it straddles the inner and outer worlds. If you think you won't be able to sleep, chances are good that you will actually have a hard time sleeping. A single thought as fleeting as *What if I'm not able to sleep tonight?* in someone who has been sensitized by a history of sleeplessness can trigger a cascade of events leading from anticipatory anxiety to increased arousal, tossing and turning in bed, acute sleep loss, and impaired daytime functioning. The situation resembles the example, often cited in discussions of chaos theory, of the butterfly whose flapping wings touch off a chain of atmospheric disturbance, ultimately unleashing hurricanes across the sea.

The skeptics among you may be wondering—if thinking can exert such direct control over sleep, why can't we just decide that we *are* able to sleep and drop right off? If sleep is so easy to obtain, why read further? In a way, your counterargument is correct. If you *truly* had confidence in your ability to sleep (and a few other conditions were met, such as your actually being sleepy), you would in fact fall asleep without difficulty. Such a scenario might be hypothetical for you, but it pretty much describes the mental state of a good sleeper.

The problem is that in your heart of hearts, you don't really believe you can readily fall asleep. Whether due to an inborn tendency toward heightened arousal, stressful life experiences, or other contributing factors, your view of going to sleep is not so straightforward. Sleep for you is not simply a response to the state of being sleepy. On the contrary, it has likely taken on all kinds of personal, idiosyncratic meanings. These meanings encrust your sleep like barnacles on a boat, impeding its progress.

In this chapter, we will see that sleep can mean very different things to different people. Whether highly prized, discounted, or dreaded, the way you think about sleep has a direct bearing on how reliably it appears. We are going to ask that you examine what sleep means to you, and if you've been finding yourself struggling at night, to consider adopting another point of view.

You are likely objecting, "I can't just change my mind like that—it's the way I think." Well, that's true to a point. But you were not born with such thoughts in your head. They got there through experience—established in reaction to events that might have occurred just in the past few months or in distant childhood. Regardless of how long they have held sway, you can challenge your beliefs about sleep if they are getting in your way. We will be guiding you toward new, more successful encounters with sleep; taking these new experiences into account should open your mind to the possibility that perhaps you are not such a hopeless case after all. Change can start right now, as you read these words, if you begin to critically examine your attitudes about sleep and at least entertain some alternative views.

A patient of ours named Sonia provides an illustration of how inhibitions over sleep are formed. We first met Sonia in her early forties, complaining of chronic difficulty falling asleep. In the course of our evaluation, we learned that unusual childhood experiences clearly shaped Sonia's attitudes toward nighttime and the process of falling asleep, attitudes which in turn helped maintain her presenting complaint.

Sonia's childhood was spent in hiding. Sequestered with a book behind the sofa or in the walk-in closet, she tried her best to be invisible, which seemed to suit her parents just fine. It wasn't physical violence that she was avoiding. That would come later, after she had run away from home. It wasn't even the yelling and screaming, although there were plenty of both, usually aimed at her siblings, who were not so adept at avoiding the line of fire. Primarily, Sonia was weathering indifference as she holed up among the shoe boxes. Her parents' ability to maintain a lifestyle that might be best described as "childless" despite having had four children continued to astound her.

Sonia and her siblings were put to bed at seven P.M., right after the dishes were cleaned. They could later hear peals of laughter from the kitchen when the McAllisters came over for cards and drinks. Sonia's younger sister didn't seem to mind the enforced bed rest. She blithely gabbed away, content with a cursory response every ten minutes or so. Sonia would read without pause, initially against her sister's drone and then in silence. Drawing upon a flashlight as the light failed, Sonia would fall asleep among the people and places circled by her beam.

Thirty years later, it was uncanny how similar her adult life was to patterns that had been set in childhood. Her primary relationships were still with characters found in books and movies. Small talk now floated across office cubicles, spouted by Sonia's fellow format specialists as their fingers glided over keyboards. After doing her best to dodge the banter, Sonia would trudge home at six P.M., bringing with her three DVDs rented for the price of two from the video store across the street. She would watch the first in her living room and the second and third from bed. Sleep would only come to her very late at night, in a bleary fade from Technicolor.

It is easy to see how Sonia's method of falling asleep established itself in childhood and later made use of changing technology. Whether escaping strife or boredom, she found comfort in the company of fiction. Unlike children who might be afraid of monsters or other imagined intruders, Sonia was most discomfited by the realities of her life. Lying in bed without diversion from these real concerns was for her an unbearable experience.

Sleep Is Meaningful

While the circumstances of Sonia's upbringing may have been un-usual, the fact that her sleeplessness was linked to personal experi-ence, that going to bed had specific *meaning* for her, is not. This is a point that is easy to overlook nowadays. It is certainly not breaking news, but rather a throwback, first to a century ago, when Freud published *The Interpretation of Dreams*, and well beyond that, to an-cient myths and religious texts in which sleep and dreams figure prominently. Going to sleep is a loaded subject. It may lead to revi-talization and to revelation, but also to missed opportunities, horren-dous accidents, and surprise attacks. On a less epic scale, the quality of our sleep determines in large part how well we feel from one day to the next.

It is a paradox that, even though we take leave of consciousness when we fall asleep, we still seem to be on intimate terms with sleep. Sleep itself may be a "black box" that remains outside our aware-ness, but the inputs and outputs of that box—what leads to sleep and what follows from it—are well known to us. In this sense of connect-ing to our waking experience, sleep does not function in obscurity as do our internal organs, nor is it so reliably automated as to practi-cally escape notice, as with much of our cognition. Because its work-ings lead to such direct and pervasive consequences for our waking lives on literally a daily basis, most of us have delved into the subject of our own sleep. We get to know its idiosyncrasies to a level of detail that would not be available if we were asked to describe, say, our kid-ney functioning, our gait, or our sense of direction. Sleep *means* a lot to us.

Having become intimately acquainted with our sleep, we all have a lot to say on the subject. This is readily apparent to those of us who work as sleep clinicians and researchers. Mention of our occupation in a social setting induces most people to give personal testimonies and judgments regarding their sleep. Usually their comments focus, in good scientific form, on the more objective, easily observable aspects of sleep: how dark the room should be, how firm the mattress, how much sleep is needed, what is likely to disrupt sleep, and which remedies are most effective at restoring it. The other topic people love to discuss is the much more subjective area of dreams.

These types of beliefs and attitudes are critically important for understanding and treating sleep disorders, but such personally meaningful information is easily overlooked in most treatment settings. This is due in part to all the progress being made in understanding the scientific underpinnings of sleep and sleeplessness—it is tempting to discount the personal, experiential dimension of sleep altogether amidst the excitement of scientific discovery.

As psychologists specializing in the treatment of insomnia, we, too, must resist the tendency to reduce sleep to its physical manifestations. Working in Sleep Disorders Centers promotes such a viewpoint. Patients who spend the night in a sleep laboratory for observation are hooked up to *polysomnographs*, machines that record electrical brain activity detected by electrodes applied across the head, as well as signals picked up by sensors monitoring changes in respiration, eye movements, muscle tone, and other functions of the body. These signals travel from the sensors down color-coded wires plugged into headboxes, through cables, and into amplifiers that produce oscillations flowing across scrolling paper or computer monitors. It is these oscillations that are scored as sleep. All these electronic gadgets in the laboratory cannot help but reflect emphasis on sleep's internal circuitry.

In the past few chapters, we have delved deep into the workings of sleep, into functional and developmental models that tell us how our bodies respond to sleep and react to the lack thereof. Let's now take a new tack and consider how you *think* about sleep. If you are unable to sleep, putting words against your problem is a very helpful first step toward resolving it.

Most of the people we see in initial consultation, when asked what has brought them in for evaluation, will say something like, "I'm not getting good sleep," "I can't get to sleep," or "I keep waking up." Fair enough—on one level these quick summaries cover most of the bases. However, sometimes our patients will not think there's much more to say. Their sleeplessness may as well have dropped from the night sky, for all it appears to relate to them. The problem does not appear to be linked, at least in their reckoning, either to past experience or current behavioral patterns and worries. We will hear, "The only thing on my mind is the fact that I'm not sleeping." Yes, that is certainly how things can look at three in the morning. However, if we are able to look a bit deeper, to help you articulate your particular relationship to sleep, to create a portrait of your sleeplessness that is closely observed and finely detailed, your prospects for regaining sleep will brighten. Let's begin with the situation, wistfully recalled by many of you we're sure, where sleep is a sought-after pleasure.

Sleep as a Pleasure

For many people, sleep is a pleasure in and of itself, ranking right up there with sex and food. People look forward to sleeping. It is a reward held out at the end of the day, motivating all kinds of toil. It may be entwined with ancillary pleasures, such as a cozy bed or a partner to snuggle with. However, sleep does not derive its worth solely from such accompaniments. Sleep is an inherent pleasure because it slakes a drive, just as surely as drink quenches a thirst. Those of you who struggle with sleep nightly may shake your heads in disbelief at this assertion, but if a typical slice of the population were asked to list their three or four greatest pleasures, "going to bed" or "sleeping in" would be a very popular choice.

If sleep is an especially treasured experience for you, its loss will be all the more debilitating. Not only are you deprived of physiological restoration, you must also bear a psychic loss. You may find yourself pining for sleep as for a lost lover. This yearning for sleep is not in your best interests. Harsh as it may seem, your prospects will improve greatly if you manage to knock sleep off its pedestal and adopt more of a "come what may" approach toward sleep accumulation. If sleep is going to play "hard to get," your best bet is cultivate a bit more indifference.

In lieu of adopting such a nonchalant attitude, you may be considering switching tacks—swearing off the pleasures of sleep, yes, but also getting on the Internet and citing all the critical functions sleep supports. However, we won't buy into your newfound health concerns. The fact is that even when you are sleeping poorly, you generally get enough sleep for basic maintenance—and perhaps even a full complement of the deep Slow Wave Sleep that is especially replenishing, given that it pushes its way to the front of the night.

Sleep as an Escape

Sleep allows a temporary getaway from the cares of the world. Insomniacs are often amazed at their friends who tend to "sleep on it" when faced with some seemingly intractable problem. "How can they act like ostriches, sticking their heads in the sand?" Their unwarranted optimism has been enshrined in such platitudes as "Go to sleep; things will look brighter in the morning." Those lucky souls who can successfully execute this strategy may be rare. However, most of us have experienced sleep as an escape under somewhat less trying circumstances, such as when we are passengers on an otherwise interminable trip. A patient of ours named Kelly, who was contending with symptoms of anxiety and depression in her waking life, was especially adept at finding refuge in bed—in case you're wondering, her presenting sleep problem was that she didn't want to get up!

Kelly felt safest when she was under the blankets. Pulling them over her head and tucking them under her feet, she didn't care whether she fell asleep or not. She recalled that even as a child, she had invested her sheets and blankets with a magical "force-field" power, able to keep the dangers of the world at bay. Kelly couldn't say for sure when this had happened. Once she had imagined that a face was peering in at the side of her bedroom window shade. Another time, she had realized with a start that a big tree towering in the backyard, viewed from just the right angle while swaying in the wind, looked just like a monster she had seen at the movies. Over time, Kelly learned that her best option for ensuring calm, given that the perils of the world outside were too powerful for her to face, was to be sure she couldn't see them.

While Kelly and the other "ostriches" who bury their heads under blankets may hardly seem like role models, we ask that you not dismiss them out of hand. Silly or not, they have come up with a way to fall asleep when dangers are pressing. Kelly's demons may have been imaginary, but her strategy (with a few twists) works surprisingly well when childhood monsters have morphed into belligerent co-workers, pending lab results, and other ravagers of adult sleep. No, you don't have to actually pull the covers over your head. An imaginary force field will do just fine. *Real problems do not have to be really solved for you to sleep.* All that is required is that you convince yourself to keep them camped outside a "problem barrier" for the night. After all, there's not much you're going to be able to do about them at two in the morning. In this respect, Kelly's cover-up strategy is quite sensible.

Another aspect of Kelly's coping strategy bears mention here: she feels safe when she climbs into bed, regardless of whether she sleeps. Her bed is her comfort. This may seem unbelievable to many of you, who are more likely to view your beds with anxiety and loathing after countless nights spent tossing and turning. Nonetheless, you should strive to get on friendly terms again with your bed, and this time on an unconditional basis—that is, not only when it manages to serve up some sleep.

Negotiating a peace treaty with your bed after months or years of struggle may strike many of you as unrealistic. We suggest that you take a step back and cast a cold eye on what each party contributed to the hostilities. Sure, if your mattress sags and your blanket itches, you would be within your rights to insist on some changes before you attempt a reconciliation. If you have spent a large part of the last three years staring at a cluster of "glow-in-the-dark" stickers or studying the dim outlines of a framed lithograph, by all means do some redecorating, so as to send a clear signal that things will be different from here on.

On the other hand, after completing your reconnaissance you may be forced to admit that your bedroom is not so bad after all. It may be that you have been unfairly maligning your bed's hospitality. Understandably, your feelings have been swayed by your experience. However, perhaps your sleeplessness stems more from the thoughts you bring into bed, or your behaviors before getting there, than from the bed itself. We encourage you to see your bed in a different light. You will come to view your bed not as a battlefield, but as snug and comfortable—a place where at the very least you can count on finding rest and respite, as well as enough sleep to get by.

Sleep as a Waste of Time

Those of us holding a particularly strong work ethic may consider sleep an indulgence or at best a pesky imposition. Slothfulness has ranked among the cardinal sins from ancient times. This attitude is reflected today among workplace managers, on the lookout for employees who have overslept slinking furtively to their desks. There is a cottage industry catering to those who would emulate Thomas Edison and function admirably on just a few hours of sleep. A patient of ours named Sid, a forty-eight-year-old public health official, was glad to hear that others were finally coming around to his point of view.

> Sid had no time for sleep. He couldn't get anything done at the office with the phone ringing all day. He had his hands full helping the kids with their homework in the evening. It was only late at night that he

could concentrate. So he improvised a bedroom office to deal with the work that inevitably overflowed home. He squeezed a desk next to the bed and topped off both dressers with milk crates holding vertical files.

Sid would work well past midnight, using his side of the bed as a staging area. He would actually have to clear a path back under the covers when he finally succumbed to exhaustion. Sometimes, he ended up sleeping next to a pile of manila envelopes rather than his wife. He would bolt upright a short while later, still an hour or two before his alarm was set to go off. Sid was amazed to think that even after his long, hectic day and his extra night shift, he still couldn't manage to fill the four or five hours he had allocated for sleep.

Our society as a whole has been subscribing to Sid's desire for quick, efficient sleep. For those who would rather produce than slumber, the Internet offers the opportunity to pursue research, pay bills, or send office e-mail in the middle of the night. A quiet household at two A.M. may well provide the best time for a busy parent to catch up on chores or paperwork. There are even more outlets available for those who would prefer to be entertained: time slots that used to be left pretty much by default to sleep are now filled with some of the most popular television talk shows. Whereas jazz clubs used to start their second set around eleven P.M., today's nightclubs have certainly not revved up and may not yet even be open at that hour.

If you are deriving too much gain after midnight, whether in pursuit of productivity or pleasure, don't expect to sleep well on "off" nights. If you are sharp enough to be polishing office presentations, alert enough to be plowing through novels, or energetic enough to go club-hopping in the middle of most nights, it is unlikely that you will be able to sleep well on a particular night just because the opportunity presents itself. If sleep is treated as "filler" material, indulged in intermittently and by default, it will return the snub.

Sleep as Letting Go

The old adage that "there will be time enough for sleeping in the grave" points to the uneasy association between sleep and death. In addition to a superficial resemblance that has figured in *Romeo and Juliet* and other literary plots, sleep requires a withdrawal of interest in the world, a loss of vigilance, and a temporary surrender to oblivion. Going to sleep becomes an act of faith. We check our identities at the threshold of sleep, on the promise that we can pick them back up on our way out. On an even more basic level, going to sleep requires trusting that we will wake up again.

Sammy felt that he had been forced into retirement by overly cautious doctors, misguided well-wishers, and inflexible Human Resources policies. Despite two heart attacks, at seventy-two, his polymer chemist's mind was still in high gear. He was a problem solver who usually did his best thinking at night. When he was working, Sammy considered these nocturnal brainstorms a boost to productivity, as welcome as a cloudburst to a farmer. He could hardly be expected to change his ways just because he had no particular assignment to complete.

His wife had informed Sammy's doctors that he was up at all hours of the night, and they had tried him on a few different sleeping medications. Initially, Sammy was intrigued with these pills, cutting them into little segments and noting the effects of various combinations, taken at various times. He designed a spreadsheet to organize his findings. None seemed all that effective. Deep down, however, Sammy knew that he was fighting the medicine. He didn't really want to go to sleep. Somehow, that would truly be conceding defeat.

Fear of losing control was clearly working against Sammy's sleep. Grappling with the physical world was central to his self-image; for him to stand down even for a few hours was no easy task. Beyond this, Sammy had lately been confronted with unmistakable harbingers of mortality, such as serious illness and forced retirement. In continuing his midnight analyses, Sammy may well have been on guard, or at least lodging a protest, against this long-term prognosis.

Good sleepers are comfortable with the process of falling asleep. They do not feel negated by sleep, but rather retain a sense of themselves throughout the experience. They enjoy drifting off and letting their minds wander over a mélange of thoughts drawn from both their everyday routines and more fantastic realms. They look forward to visiting dreamscapes and readily make connections between events occurring within their dreams and those from waking life. Overall, they do not feel that sleep lies on the far side of a chasm that has to somehow be surmounted nightly. For comfortable sleepers, sleep is a native land, with a geography and language they understand.

Clearing Your Mind for Sleep

Some of you may be dealing with feelings similar to Sammy's. You end up repelling sleep because you are afraid you might lose yourself in it. You find yourself comforted by that familiar internal voice that keeps up a running commentary on the outside world from its command post in your darkened bedroom. You come to believe that your very identity is wrapped up in that voice. Its opinions, biases, fears, memories—it is *who you are*. Its ongoing patter reassures you even as it prevents you from drifting off to sleep. This inner voice is proof of your existence, a nightly demonstration of the Cartesian premise "I think, therefore I am."

Paradoxically, the optimal mind-set for sleep is mindlessness. When it comes to sleeping, the mind is a bit of a bumbler, getting in its own way. Ideally, if we're thinking at all at the end of a full day, it should be about how tired we are and how much we are going to enjoy climbing into bed. Sleepiness should render both our concerns and our enthusiasms increasingly tepid. The desired effect should be one of a slow fade-out, where hard-edged recollections of the day dissolve into flowing reveries before consciousness is finally lost.

Nature's script may call for an imperceptible segue, and such a transition may characterize the experience of the best sleepers. But the majority of brains do not give up the ghost so easily. As with HAL, the wayward computer in *2001: A Space Odyssey*; Sammy the pill splitter; or, closer to home, the typical three-year-old resisting bedtime, most of us seem to dread shutting down. Our minds will alight on any available perch, be it an innocuous jingle, a vexing memory, or a perceived threat, rather than slip into the void.

You are, therefore, likely inclined to harbor your inner news anchor as tenaciously as a three-year-old clutches her teddy bear. Nonetheless, if you wish to sleep well, this assertive commentator must yield to a passive listener, a swamilike soul who registers any and all events with equanimity. You must be willing not to care, not to protest, not to stand up as an individual and be counted—at least until morning. You must relinquish control, not only over whatever may come your way from the world outside your bedroom as you sleep, but also over *your own thoughts*—over the reveries and dreams contrived by your sleepy and sleeping mind.

Easy enough to say, you're probably thinking, *but not so easy to accomplish when the night is already getting short and anxiety is welling up like floodwater*. We are confident you will in fact soon be able to let go, to detach yourself from sleep. Having just expounded on the power of the mind to forestall sleep, how can we be so sure? Well, you have an ally in this effort who has gone unappreciated, whose talents for slumber have not been put to full use. What ally? Your physiology—your body. Recall for a moment those times when, after a long string of awful nights, you just physically collapsed. It finally did not matter what was on your mind; sleep just overwhelmed you. Your limbs went heavy; your breathing slowed; your eyelids tugged down. You were going to sleep, no matter what.

We are not suggesting that this is the right way to fall asleep—every third or fourth night, only out of sheer exhaustion. This, after all, is probably the way you are sleeping now! However, our example does highlight the enormous potential for sleep contained within your body. In the second part of this book, we show you how to harness this physiological pull into sleep, how to couple it to a tranquil mind, and how to mete it out on a nightly basis. We start by reciting an alphabet of sleep, a simple litany that will prep you for slumber.

PART TWO

The ABCDEs of Sleep

Congratulations! You now have a broad understanding of the physical and psychological mechanisms that help us sleep, as well as those that keep us awake. This knowledge will provide a strong foundation on which to build a reliable sleep/wake cycle. Now we are ready to add information about *your* insomnia, gleaned from the responses you will provide on a few short questionnaires, as well as from a one-week baseline sleep log. With this data in hand, we will be able to prescribe a simple "Preliminary Treatment," tailored to your sleep pattern. This initial treatment should noticeably moderate your insomnia, regardless of the exact nature of the problems you have been facing. Moreover, it will prime your mind and body for sleep, enhancing the effectiveness of subsequent interventions.

After the Preliminary Treatment phase, we will direct you to interventions that target the particular sleep disturbance you are contending with. As you have learned, insomnia can result from a wide array of interacting factors. Once triggered, it can manifest itself in a wide range of patterns. Most succinctly, insomnia can do the bulk of its damage to the beginning of the night, it can riddle the entire span of your sleep with holes, or it can bring your night to a premature end. Within each of these broad groupings, a number of insomnia subtypes can be seen. It would be unlikely that such a protean adversary could be subdued with a single treatment. By analyzing your sleep pattern in greater detail and taking more of its contributing factors into account, we will be able to guide you through an optimally personalized treatment strategy.

Once you set the stage for better sleep with our Preliminary Treatment and then apply treatments specifically targeting your type of insomnia, what could stand in the way of improvement? The answer to this question will probably not come as a surprise: *you yourself* may still need convincing that sleep will show up on schedule; otherwise its appearance may indeed be delayed or canceled. As we have seen, these last-minute internal negotiations can be touchy. If you are afraid of lowering your level of vigilance, if you don't have confidence in your ability to sleep, if you are too worried about the consequences of losing sleep—even if you sabotage yourself on a whim, for no reason at all—your sleep may balk. Therefore, in our closing chapter, we reconvene you all as a group and show you how to disengage your mind, how to cease resistance, and how to allow yourself to drift off on a wave of sleep.

Generally, early interventions will remain in place as others are added. Our approach involves a cascade of treatments, each addressing different aspects of your insomnia, moving you progressively closer to your objective of deep, reliable sleep. We ask your indulgence if you have already tried some components of our program in the past, without seeing much benefit. If a three-legged table falls over, it's not the fault of the existing legs; the problem lies with what's missing. You will need to assemble a complete treatment regimen, and gain the confidence that comes from increasing success, before your sleep is fully stabilized. This may sound a bit daunting. But in truth it's as straightforward as ABC. Here are the demands sleep will be making of you, before it strikes a deal to appear nightly.

Address Your Insomnia Factors

The first step in your Preliminary Treatment program is to deal with, as best you can, any issues you are able to identify as intruding on your sleep. We say "as best you can" because, as you learned in Chapter 3, these likely include some causes that are difficult to avoid completely. For example, you may have been predisposed to sleep disturbance by a long-standing history of depression. Or your insomnia might have been precipitated by losing your job. Even in these cases, you can take actions to at least improve your prospects for sleep. Perhaps you have been putting off seeking treatment for symptoms of mood disturbance. Now is the time to bring up these concerns with your doctor. Perhaps you have been spinning your wheels in the search for a new job. Now is the time to join a networking group or consult a placement specialist. We fully understand that some problems contributing to insomnia can be tenacious. They certainly will not be resolved in a night. However, taking specific action aimed at the eventual resolution of these problems is critical—it will allow you to "sign off" on today's efforts and marshal your resources for tomorrow's challenges.

The most common problems sustaining insomnia—even in cases where Predisposing characteristics such as depression and Precipitating events such as job loss initially loomed large—are Perpetuating attitudes and practices that develop in response to sleeplessness. For example, sleep hygiene breaks down amidst our efforts to counteract poor sleep. Thus, we start oversleeping on weekends, get into the habit of reading in bed during the middle of the night, or begin relying too heavily on caffeine to get through the day. Fortunately, once targeted, these maladaptive responses can be reversed quickly, bringing rapid improvement in sleep.

Boost Your Sleep Drive

Second, you will need to have an adequate Sleep Drive at the moment your head hits the pillow. Achieving this is not complicated—as should be recalled from Chapter 2, you simply must remain wakeful long enough and let homeostasis do the rest. However, just because a task is straightforward doesn't mean it will be easy. This fact was clearly appreciated by the philosopher Friedrich Nietzsche, who wrote:

> *No small art is it to sleep; for its sake must one stay awake all day.*

How long is long enough to stay awake? The answer to this fundamental question will differ for each of you, depending upon the strength of your Sleep Drive, as well as the intensity of the Alerting Force that opposes it. We can get a sense of your current propensity for sleep by charting the amount of sleep you actually accumulate, relative to the bedtime you set aside for obtaining it. You will shortly be filling out a sleep log to do just that.

Choose the Right Time for Bed

The third step, which completes your Preliminary Treatment, is to choose a bedtime that occurs at an appropriate position along the falling slope of the circadian Alerting Force rhythm. If your bedtime is too close to the peak of this rhythm, your body will not yet be ready to sleep. If your bedtime is positioned too far down along the slope, your circadian physiology will begin to push you toward wakefulness prematurely, after just a few hours of sleep. Going to bed at the right time will ensure that the Alerting Force continues to di-

---

PRELIMINARY TREATMENT RATIONALE

Address Your Insomnia Factors

Boost Your Sleep Drive

Choose the Right Time for Bed

Enhance your chances of sleeping well by first removing obstacles to sleep: improve poor sleep hygiene, treat depression, counter hyperarousal, cease worrying about sleep, and instead take on the role of a neutral observer.

Then recruit the two fundamental processes regulating sleep to work on your behalf: increase your homeostatic drive for sleep, and schedule your bedtime to coincide with the hours when you are most likely to fall asleep and stay asleep. This will help you fall asleep more quickly and maintain deeper, more consolidated sleep.

minish throughout almost the entire night and that you will garner an adequate amount of sleep.

Precisely locating the peak and trough of the Alerting Force is not something that can be done easily at home. Fortunately, there are ways of estimating where these points are. For now, the easiest way to approximate the location of the trough of your circadian Alerting Force is simply to determine which block of hours in the day or night you are most likely to sleep through when selecting your own schedule. The sleep log you will soon be keeping will also enable you to find these optimal hours for sleep.

Differentiate Your Therapy

When you have addressed as best you can the factors impeding your sleep, boosted your sleep drive by shortening the amount of time you spend in bed, and chosen a bedtime that aligns with your circadian propensity for sleep, it will be time to tailor your treatment to the specific type of insomnia that plagues you. Some treatments are geared toward those who have difficulty falling asleep, some toward those who have trouble staying asleep, and some toward those whose sleep is broken by many awakenings or who have no discernable sleep pattern at all.

Ease Your Mind

The final condition for entering sleep, regardless of the particular nature of your insomnia and the specific remedies you apply, is to be able to withdraw your interest from the external world and from your own thoughts as well. You must manage to find neutral mental territory, a vantage point from which issues and concerns receive passing acknowledgment but register no real impact. Many people with insomnia liken their minds at bedtime to a speeding train that they cannot stop. They exert themselves mightily in what is often a futile attempt to apply the brakes. If you find yourself in this situation, it's best to amble back to a passenger seat and simply look out the window. Yes, there are interesting and even menacing things out there, but they will pass in the night if you can cultivate an attitude of detachment.

You must make your peace with the events of the day just past, feel secure in your bed, and achieve a degree of equanimity regarding the challenges you will face tomorrow. As we discussed in Chapter 4, you must become cognizant of the way you think about sleep itself, because your attitudes and beliefs about sleep will either facilitate or impede its appearance. Achieving tranquility is a tall order, one that is best not attempted in a rush. Rather, the process of easing your mind into sleep should begin as soon as you start your day. You will need to feel satisfied with your entire day's accomplishments to successfully negotiate its end. Nietzsche apparently knew this as well:

Ten truths must you find during the day; otherwise, will you seek truth during the night...

CHAPTER FIVE

Preliminary Treatment

Identifying Which Type of Insomnia
You Have and Preparing Yourself
for Better Sleep

Now that you understand what makes for a good night's sleep, as well as how sleep can go awry, it's time to treat your insomnia. First, we need to investigate issues that may be inclining you to insomnia or maintaining your sleeplessness. These factors should be addressed before we begin building waves of sleep and positioning you to catch them nightly. We will gather the information we need via a few simple questionnaires and a basic Sleep Log, which you'll use to record your sleep for a week.

Address Your Insomnia Factors

Start by completing the Insomnia Symptom Questionnaire and the Fatigue Severity Scale on the following pages. These scales will assess your current level of sleep disturbance and fatigue. They will not direct your treatment but rather allow you to gauge your progress—we will return to them in about a month to see how you are doing!

The remaining questionnaires and the Sleep Log will be found just ahead of the sections in which they are discussed. Scoring guidelines for all scales and questionnaires are presented in the Endnotes section pertaining to this chapter. When you fill out the Sleep Hygiene Awareness and Practices Questionnaire, err on the side of inclusion as you try to identify practices that could conceivably bear on your sleep problem. Do not prejudge whether a given practice is personally relevant. We want you to assume that they all are and address each one! The Zung Self-Rating Depression Scale broadly surveys symptoms of this complex disorder. Scores higher than fifty-nine indicate increasing likelihood that significant depression is present and playing some role in maintaining your insomnia.

The Pre-Sleep Arousal Scale assesses aspects of physiological and cognitive hyperarousal that may inhibit the arrival of sleep. The endorsement of several items on this scale indicates that hyperarousal is more likely to be a factor predisposing you to sleeplessness. However, if just one manifestation of hyperarousal is present in sufficient intensity, sleep can suffer. The same can be said for the Dysfunctional Beliefs and Attitudes About Sleep scale. It can serve as a checklist, helping you recognize views you may be harboring that are counterproductive to sleep. Just one such belief or attitude will unnecessarily raise the stakes and thereby render sleep more of a gamble.

INSOMNIA SYMPTOM QUESTIONNAIRE

NEVER	N
RARELY	R
SOMETIMES	S
FREQUENTLY	F
ALWAYS	A

Patient: _____

Day: _____ Date: _____ Time: _____

Answer the following questions based on the <u>previous 7 days</u>.

1. Do you lie awake at night worried, anxious or distressed?   N R S F A

2. During the day do you worry about how you will sleep that night?   N R S F A

3. Are you watching the clock or aware of time passing while lying awake in bed?   N R S F A

4. Is your sleep restless?   N R S F A

5. Are you experiencing <u>brief</u> awakenings during the night?   N R S F A

6. Are you experiencing <u>long</u> awakenings during the night?   N R S F A

7. Do you feel tired or fatigued during the day or evening?   N R S F A

8. Have you taken any naps or fallen asleep briefly during the day or evening?   N R S F A

9. Have you been sleepy or drowsy during the day or evening?   N R S F A

10. Do you feel you have been getting an adequate amount of sleep?   N R S F A

11. Do you feel you have been getting good quality sleep?   N R S F A

12. Since the last time you answered this questionnaire is your sleep now . . .
   Much Better   Better   No Different   Worse   Much Worse

FATIGUE SEVERITY SCALE

This scale contains nine statements relating to fatigue and its consequences. Read each statement and circle a number from 1 to 7, depending on how well you feel the statement applies to you, judging from the preceding week. A low value indicates that the statement hardly applies to you, whereas a high value indicates that the statement applies very well.

During the past week, I have found that: **Score**

1. My motivation is lower when I am fatigued.   1 2 3 4 5 6 7

2. Exercise brings on my fatigue.   1 2 3 4 5 6 7

3. I am easily fatigued.   1 2 3 4 5 6 7

4. Fatigue interferes with my physical functioning.   1 2 3 4 5 6 7

5. Fatigue causes frequent problems for me.   1 2 3 4 5 6 7

6. My fatigue prevents sustained physical functioning.   1 2 3 4 5 6 7

7. Fatigue interferes with carrying out certain duties
    and responsibilities.   1 2 3 4 5 6 7

8. Fatigue is among my three most disabling symptoms. 1 2 3 4 5 6 7

9. Fatigue interferes with my work, family, or social life. 1 2 3 4 5 6 7

Score by calculating the average response to the questions (adding up all the answers and dividing by nine).

ADDRESS YOUR INSOMNIA FACTORS
EVALUATION PHASE

Insomnia Symptom Questionnaire
Assess your insomnia before and after starting our program so you can track your progress.

Fatigue Severity Scale
Assess your fatigue level before and after starting our program.

Sleep Hygiene Awareness and Practices
Identify activities and practices of everyday living that may be obstacles to better sleep.

Zung Self-Rating Depression Scale
Assess the potential contribution of depression to your sleep problem.

Pre-Sleep Arousal Scale
Gauge the level of your overactivation.

Dysfunctional Beliefs and Attitudes About Sleep
Survey your counterproductive thinking about sleeplessness.

Sleep Logs
Log your time in bed, your sleep, and periods of wakefulness. This will help in analyzing your sleep problem, tailoring your treatment, and tracking your progress.

SLEEP HYGIENE AWARENESS AND PRACTICES

For each of the following behaviors state the number of days per week (0-7) that you engage in that activity or have that experience. Base your answers on what you would consider an *average* week for yourself.

Indicate the number of days or nights in an average week you:

1. Take a nap _____
2. Go to bed hungry _____
3. Go to bed thirsty _____
4. Smoke cigarettes _____
5. Use sleeping medications (prescription or over-the-counter) _____
6. Drink beverages containing caffeine (e.g., coffee, tea, colas) after noon _____
7. Drink alcohol within 3 hours of bedtime _____
8. Take medications/drugs with caffeine within 4 hours of bedtime _____
9. Worry as you prepare for bed about your ability to sleep _____
10. Worry during the day about your ability to sleep at night _____
11. Use alcohol to facilitate sleep _____
12. Exercise strenuously within 2 hours of bedtime _____
13. Have your sleep disturbed by light _____
14. Have your sleep disturbed by noise _____
15. Have your sleep disturbed by your bedpartner _____ (put NA if no partner)
16. Sleep approximately the same length of time each night _____
17. Set aside time to relax before bedtime _____
18. Exercise in the afternoon or early evening _____
19. Have a comfortable night-time temperature in your bed/bedroom _____

IMPROVE YOUR SLEEP HYGIENE

We suggested at the outset of this book that you attend to your sleep hygiene. For a few lucky readers, these basic recommendations may have been enough to set sleep aright. Those of you still reading will need to add more focused treatments to your sleep regimen. Even so, as we begin the next phase of our work together, take a hard-eyed look at your responses on the recently completed Sleep Hygiene Awareness and Practices questionnaire. It is very common for people with insomnia to overlook proper sleep hygiene because they believe the recommendations don't really apply to them. They maintain that they can drink coffee with impunity, nap as they please, or sleep with all three of their dogs probably because they have learned through experience that their sleep is a mess whether they do so or not. The belief that you are somehow immune to sleep hygiene requirements is dysfunctional. We will soon be applying some powerful new therapies in the cause of improving your sleep—now is the time to do everything in your power to help these treatments help you.

Some of the suggestions will be relatively easy to comply with. For example, you may just need to follow through on that notion to purchase blackout curtains for your bedroom, or a fan, or a white noise generator. However, other sleep hygiene recommendations are much harder to implement. Oftentimes, they ask you to deny yourself something, whether a nap or a nightcap, that feels good and brings at least short-term relief.

You stand a better chance of maintaining proper sleep hygiene if you take control over the dispensing of these indulgences, rather than having them triggered by external influences. For example, your daily coffee consumption may work out to eight cups because each cup is associated with a particular situation: two cups at breakfast, one when you get into work, another on your morning break, etc. If you don't make a conscious decision to limit caffeine and have a plan in place to effect this change, you will continue to drink about eight cups per day for the foreseeable future. If you find yourself in this situation, draw up a schedule that allocates seven cups of coffee across the day for a week or so, then six cups, and so on. Don't rely on a vague idea that you just need to "cut down." If you decide to forego the cup that usually greets you when you first arrive at work, what are you going to replace it with?

An alternative strategy that will allow you to cut back on caffeine is to manipulate the strength of the brew. Initially, you might brew full-strength coffee at home with breakfast and switch to half-decaffeinated coffee later in the day. After a week or so, you will want to change your evening coffee entirely to a decaffeinated blend, and gradually replace most or all of your daily consumption with decaffeinated coffee, working back toward morning.

If you nap two or more times a day, this may indicate that the continuity of your sleep is being repeatedly broken by some kind of physiological disturbance such as sleep-disordered breathing or periodic limb movements. These conditions will likely require specialized testing to evaluate. People suffering from insomnia are actually less likely to nap because they tend toward hyperarousal, both during the day and the night. However, some insomnia sufferers do nap during the day. If your sleep appears to be of adequate quality but insufficient quantity (at least at night), you may require a daytime nap until your nocturnal sleep is better consolidated. However, again it will be important for you to take charge of your sleep hygiene rather than napping whenever the opportunity presents itself. Work toward a target of just one nap in the early afternoon, limited to about half an hour, if you hope to sleep through the bulk of the night. Get in the habit of setting an alarm clock when you lie down to prevent oversleeping.

You should adopt a similarly firm and active stance toward revising any other sleep hygiene deficiencies you have identified. If you habitually doze in front of the television in the evening and then have trouble falling asleep later that night, the fact that your dozing is inadvertent is no excuse. Don't be so sedentary or make yourself so comfortable after dinner. Save the TV viewing and the easy chair for late in the evening, when the sleepiness they induce can be put to good effect. It may indeed be too late to banish your eight-year-old retriever from the bed, short of fashioning a spiked coverlet. But there may still be time to retrain a young dog to at least sleep on a floor cushion, if not in another room.

ZUNG SELF-RATING DEPRESSION SCALE

Name: _____ Date: _____

Please read each statement and decide how much of the time the statement describes how you have been feeling during the past several days.

Make a check mark (✓) in appropriate column.

	A little of the time	Some of the time	Good part of the time	Most of the time
1. I feel down-hearted and blue				
2. Morning is when I feel the best				
3. I have crying spells or feel like it				
4. I have trouble sleeping at night				
5. I eat as much as I used to				
6. I still enjoy sex				
7. I notice that I am losing weight				
8. I have trouble with constipation				
9. My heart beats faster than usual				
10. I get tired for no reason				
11. My mind is as clear as it used to be				
12. I find it easy to do the things I used to				
13. I am restless and can't keep still				
14. I feel hopeful about the future				
15. I am more irritable than usual				
16. I find it easy to make decisions				
17. I feel that I am useful and needed				
18. My life is pretty full				
19. I feel that others would be better off if I were dead				
20. I still enjoy the things I used to do				

Adapted from Zung, A self-rating depression scale, *Arch Gen Psychiatry*, 1965;12:63–70.

SEEK TREATMENT FOR YOUR DEPRESSION

If your Zung score is moderately or severely elevated, it's probably not telling you anything you don't already know—it was you, after all, who supplied the responses. The main contribution of such an assessment is really just to give a name to your collection of symptoms. However, this is of no small importance. You would be surprised at how many people are ready to acknowledge that they have been withdrawn and apathetic of late, feeling somewhat blue, a bit tearful, and without appetite for sex or food—but still reluctant to consider that they are suffering from depression. Even their doctors may share this tendency to overlook the presence of depression if it is not explicitly presented as a concern, in the press to cover physical complaints.

Depression not only has a direct bearing on sleep architecture and sleep quality—a major reason why we have singled it out for detection in our assessment battery—it also saps motivation for change, making compliance with treatment recommendations much more difficult. The good news is that there are numerous effective pharmacological and cognitive-behavioral treatments for depression. If you are suffering from depression, we urge you to consult with your doctor regarding a course of treatment. Your efforts at improving both mood and sleep can run in parallel so that no time will be lost, and they will in fact enhance each other's prospects for success.

Some cases of insomnia will resolve directly upon treatment of an underlying depression; others will not. However, concurrent treatment of depression will let the insomnia answers presented in this book bring you maximum benefit. If on the other hand, your depression goes undetected or is acknowledged but allowed to fester, you may follow our instructions regarding sleep interventions to the letter without perceiving much improvement.

PRE-SLEEP AROUSAL

Name: _____ Date: _____

During the pre-sleep period last night (in bed with the lights out before falling asleep for the first time), did you have any of the following experiences? Please indicate (by circling the approprate number) the degree to which you experienced each of those listed below. Do not include what you experienced during the middle of the night if you awakened after falling asleep.

	Not at all	A little	Moderately	A lot	Extremely
1. Heart racing, pounding, or beating irregularly	1	2	3	4	5
2. A jittery, nervous feeling in your body	1	2	3	4	5
3. Worry about falling asleep	1	2	3	4	5
4. Review or ponder events of the day	1	2	3	4	5
5. Shortness of breath or labored breathing	1	2	3	4	5
6. Depressing or anxious thoughts	1	2	3	4	5
7. A tight, tense feeling in your muscles	1	2	3	4	5
8. Worry about problems other than sleep	1	2	3	4	5
9. Being mentally alert, active	1	2	3	4	5
10. Cold feeling in your hands, feet, or your body in general	1	2	3	4	5
11. Can't shut off your thoughts	1	2	3	4	5
12. Have stomach upset (knot or nervous feeling in stomach, heartburn, nausea, gas, etc.)	1	2	3	4	5
13. Perpsiration in palms of your hands or other parts of your body	1	2	3	4	5
14. Thoughts keep running through your head	1	2	3	4	5
15. Dry feeling in mouth or throat	1	2	3	4	5
16. Distracted by sounds, noise in the environment (e.g, ticking clock, house noises, traffic)	1	2	3	4	5

COUNTER HYPERAROUSAL WITH EXERCISE, BEHAVIOR THERAPY, OR PHARMACOLOGIC TREATMENTS

We have discussed the fact that hyperarousal is a characteristic commonly predisposing people to insomnia, so you should not be surprised if you endorsed a high number of items on the Pre-Sleep Arousal Scale. As with depression, a number of pharmacologic and nonpharmacologic treatments are available to counter hyperarousal. Indeed, many of you are coming to this treatment while on medications that serve to ease anxiety or promote sedation. As explained at the outset, if you are on such medication, we suggest that you try to implement the behavioral and cognitive treatments in this book before consulting with your doctor about possibly tapering the dosage. However, if you are not currently using medication and are not in crisis, we ask that you avoid taking such drugs while you put our recommendations into practice. Oftentimes, making room in your schedule for such activities as regular exercise, yoga classes, or stress-management workshops will effectively address hyperarousal and set the stage for better sleep.

While both depression and hyperarousal often lead to insomnia, we prioritize the treatment of these two Predisposing factors differently. We encourage you to address depression directly and independently of the treatments you will be following to bolster your sleep. With regard to hyperarousal, however, we will be addressing this risk factor for insomnia within the general regimen set up to improve your sleep. We take this route partly because of the differing natures of these conditions and their associated risks, partly because the drug treatments that address hyperarousal are prone to the development of tolerance (so that higher doses are often required with long-term use), and partly because a number of the behavioral interventions we will be introducing have a specific action, whether direct or indirect, against hyperarousal.

DYSFUNCTIONAL BELIEFS AND ATTITUDES ABOUT SLEEP (DBAS)

Name: _____ Date: _____

Several statements reflecting people's beliefs and attitudes about sleep are listed below. Please indicate to what extent you personally agree or disagree with each statement. There is no right or wrong answer. For each statement, circle the number that corresponds to your own *personal belief*. Please respond to all items even though some may not apply directly to your own situation.

Strongly   Strongly
Disagree   Agree

0   1   2   3   4   5   6   ⑦   8   9   10

1. I need 8 hours of sleep to feel refreshed and function well during the day.

    0   1   2   3   4   5   6   7   8   9   10

2. When I don't get a proper amount of sleep on a given night, I need to catch up on the next day by napping or on the next night by sleeping longer.

    0   1   2   3   4   5   6   7   8   9   10

3. Because I am getting older, I need less sleep.

    0   1   2   3   4   5   6   7   8   9   10

4. I am worried that if I go for 1 or 2 nights without sleep, I may have a "nervous breakdown."

    0   1   2   3   4   5   6   7   8   9   10

5. I am concerned that chronic insomnia may have serious consequences for my physical health.

    0   1   2   3   4   5   6   7   8   9   10

Strongly Disagree										Strongly Agree
0	1	2	3	4	5	6	⑦	8	9	10

6. By spending more time in bed, I usually get more sleep and feel better the next day.

0	1	2	3	4	5	6	7	8	9	10

7. When I have trouble falling asleep or getting back to sleep after nighttime awakening, I should stay in bed and try harder.

0	1	2	3	4	5	6	7	8	9	10

8. I am worried that I may lose control over my abilities to sleep.

0	1	2	3	4	5	6	7	8	9	10

9. Because I am getting older, I should go to bed earlier in the evening.

0	1	2	3	4	5	6	7	8	9	10

10. After a poor night's sleep, I know that it will interfere with my daily activities on the next day.

0	1	2	3	4	5	6	7	8	9	10

11. In order to be alert and function well during the day, I believe I would be better off taking a sleeping pill rather than having a poor night's sleep.

0	1	2	3	4	5	6	7	8	9	10

12. When I feel irritable, depressed, or anxious during the day, it is mostly because I did not sleep well the night before.

0	1	2	3	4	5	6	7	8	9	10

Strongly
Disagree

0	1	2	3	4	5	6	(7)	8	9	10

Strongly
Agree

13. Because my bed partner falls asleep as soon as his/her head hits the pillow and stays asleep through the night, I should be able to do so too.

0	1	2	3	4	5	6	7	8	9	10

14. I feel that insomnia is basically the result of aging and there isn't much that can be done about this problem.

0	1	2	3	4	5	6	7	8	9	10

15. I am sometimes afraid of dying in my sleep.

0	1	2	3	4	5	6	7	8	9	10

16. When I have a good night's sleep, I know that I will have to pay for it on the following night.

0	1	2	3	4	5	6	7	8	9	10

17. When I sleep poorly on one night, I know it will disturb my sleep schedule for the whole week.

0	1	2	3	4	5	6	7	8	9	10

18. Without an adequate night's sleep, I can hardly function the next day.

0	1	2	3	4	5	6	7	8	9	10

19. I can't ever predict whether I'll have a good or poor night's sleep.

0	1	2	3	4	5	6	7	8	9	10

Strongly
Disagree

Strongly
Agree

| 0 | 1 | 2 | 3 | 4 | 5 | 6 | (7) | 8 | 9 | 10 |

20. I have little ability to manage the negative consequences of disturbed sleep.

| 0 | 1 | 2 | 3 | 4 | 5 | 6 | 7 | 8 | 9 | 10 |

21. When I feel tired, have no energy, or just seem not to function well during the day, it is generally because I did not sleep well the night before.

| 0 | 1 | 2 | 3 | 4 | 5 | 6 | 7 | 8 | 9 | 10 |

22. I get overwhelmed by my thoughts at night and often feel I have no control over this racing mind.

| 0 | 1 | 2 | 3 | 4 | 5 | 6 | 7 | 8 | 9 | 10 |

23. I feel I can still lead a satisfactory life despite sleep difficulties.

| 0 | 1 | 2 | 3 | 4 | 5 | 6 | 7 | 8 | 9 | 10 |

24. I believe insomnia is essentially the result of a chemical imbalance.

| 0 | 1 | 2 | 3 | 4 | 5 | 6 | 7 | 8 | 9 | 10 |

25. I feel insomnia is ruining my ability to enjoy life and prevents me from doing what I want.

| 0 | 1 | 2 | 3 | 4 | 5 | 6 | 7 | 8 | 9 | 10 |

26. A "nightcap" before bedtime is a good solution to sleep problems.

| 0 | 1 | 2 | 3 | 4 | 5 | 6 | 7 | 8 | 9 | 10 |

27. Medication is probably the only solution to sleeplessness.

| 0 | 1 | 2 | 3 | 4 | 5 | 6 | 7 | 8 | 9 | 10 |

Strongly Disagree										**Strongly Agree**
0	1	2	3	4	5	6	⑦	8	9	10

28. My sleep is getting worse all the time and I don't believe anyone can help.

0	1	2	3	4	5	6	7	8	9	10

29. It usually shows in my physical appearance when I haven't slept well.

0	1	2	3	4	5	6	7	8	9	10

30. I avoid or cancel obligations (social, family) after a poor night's sleep.

0	1	2	3	4	5	6	7	8	9	10

QUESTION YOUR BELIEFS ABOUT SLEEP

Inspection of your responses on the Dysfunctional Beliefs and Attitudes About Sleep Scale may indicate that some of your ideas about sleep are inaccurate and counterproductive. These misguided beliefs raise the stakes with regard to getting to sleep, making that prospect even less likely. Of course, if you really hold dearly to the notion that you need more than ten hours of sleep to function at all the next day, just hearing from us that this is implausible will probably not prompt a change of mind. You may insist you are the highly unusual case, the one in a thousand who requires that much sleep! We must agree that, with the normal distribution of habitual sleep time ranging between six and nine hours, there are bound to be a few outliers in either direction who have more extreme requirements. However, "long sleepers" do just that—they sleep a long time, consistently. Your chronic difficulty getting to sleep or staying asleep argues strongly against your inclusion in this group.

Logic aside, what really is required is a demonstration that you do better with six, seven, or eight hours of sleep consolidated into a shorter bedtime than when you stretch sleep thin, trying to cover nine or ten hours in bed. Until this can be accomplished, we ask you to open your mind to the possibility that your sleep needs may not be so unusual, that perhaps your sleep mechanisms are not broken, that you are in fact susceptible to the alerting effects of caffeine or the disruptive effects of alcohol—that in general, the practices that work well for good sleepers may bring you benefits also.

ADDRESS YOUR INSOMNIA FACTORS

Your **Insomnia Assessment Battery** will suggest a number of changes you should make in your behavior and thinking. While these changes may not in themselves lead to reliable sleep, they will set the stage for effective treatment.

Improve Your Sleep Hygiene
- Set regular times for retiring to and arising from bed.
- Limit oversleeping on weekends.
- Refrain from daytime naps and momentary dozing.
- Allow sufficient time to wind down before bedtime.
- Discontinue all alcohol, and taper off caffeine.
- Limit fluids in the evening.
- Do not look at your clock at night.
- Keep your room dark and quiet.
- Be sure your bed partner or pet is not disturbing your sleep.

Seek Treatment for Depression
- You will be more likely to improve your sleep, and to maintain your progress, if you directly address depression while you are dealing with your insomnia.

Counter Hyperarousal with Behavioral or Pharmacologic Treatments
- Employ exercise, relaxation, meditation, or "time-outs" daily to address cognitive and physiological hyperarousal. Use what has worked best for you in the past.
- If you are presently using sedating or hypnotic medications, remain on the regimen you have worked out with your doctor for the time being.

Question Your Beliefs About Sleep
- Do not fuel your insomnia through worry; for the next month or two, try to suspend your judgment as to how much sleep you need, how you will be able to function without sleep, the effects of insomnia on your health and mood, whether the treatment will work, and so on. Try to adopt a more distanced, neutral stance with regard to your sleep.

Boost Your Sleep Drive

In addition to addressing the factors behind your insomnia, there is a second way in which you can achieve more reliable sleep: you could directly strengthen your Sleep Drive. Suppose you wanted to improve railroad service across a high mountain pass. You could work on the track, perhaps re-grading steeper stretches that have been slowing down the trains. This would be akin to smoothing out the path toward sleep by improving sleep hygiene or addressing other insomnia factors. However, there are also gains to be made by simply hitching up to a more powerful locomotive. In this section, we will show you how to turbocharge your Sleep Drive.

To do so, we will need to analyze how your sleep is currently operating. We will need to get a sense of its efficiency—how well your sleep fills up its available bedtime. We also will want to gauge when across the night and day your sleep is most robust, and when it appears to be most in need of a boost. We can accomplish these critical diagnostic tasks with a Sleep Log.

START YOUR SLEEP LOG

Many people with insomnia believe that their sleep is totally random. They object to the need to fill out a Sleep Log, arguing that there is no pattern to depict. This perception is understandable. As we contend with chronic sleep problems, our cycles do in fact tend to break down, with more variability appearing in bedtimes and rising times, and more napping interspersed across the week. However, most insomniacs have some residual sleep/wake pattern. This pattern may indeed be hard to see from a night-to-night vantage point, but it will

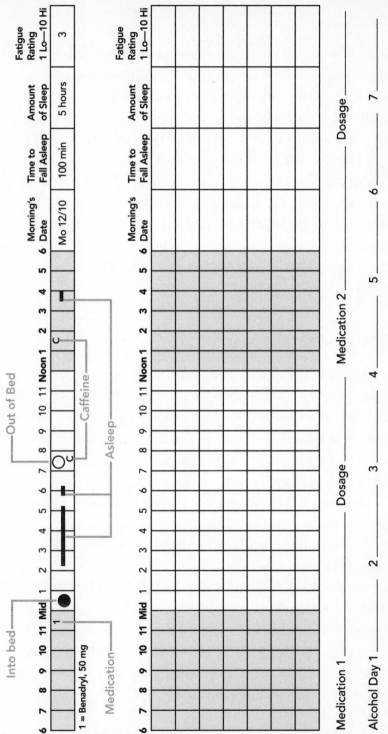

Into bed —

Out of Bed —

6	7	8	9	10	11	Mid	1	2	3	4	5	6	7	8	9	10	11	Noon	1	2	3	4	5	6 Morning's Date	Time to Fall Asleep	Amount of Sleep	Fatigue Rating 1 Lo—10 Hi

Mo 12/10 | 100 min | 5 hours | 3

Medication

1 = Benadryl, 50 mg

Caffeine

Asleep

| 6 | 7 | 8 | 9 | 10 | 11 | Mid | 1 | 2 | 3 | 4 | 5 | 6 | 7 | 8 | 9 | 10 | 11 | Noon | 1 | 2 | 3 | 4 | 5 | 6 Morning's Date | Time to Fall Asleep | Amount of Sleep | Fatigue Rating 1 Lo—10 Hi |

Medication 1 _____ Dosage _____

Medication 2 _____ Dosage _____

Alcohol Day 1 ___ 2 ___ 3 ___ 4 ___ 5 ___ 6 ___ 7 ___

come into focus if you track your sleep over a string of nights. It helps to take a longer view—just as geographical features may be lost at ground level, yet clearly spied from an airplane. If you find yourself lying in bed wondering where your sleep has gone and when it is likely to return, it would behoove you to do more than just pass the time in idle speculation. You should begin filling out a Sleep Log.

We designed a log some years ago, reproduced on the previous page for your use, which can help you discern the remnants of any pattern that might remain in your tattered sleep. It allows you to illustrate an entire week on one page, and it uses a small number of symbols and graphic conventions to depict key features of your sleep experience.

HOW TO COMPLETE YOUR LOG

A sample night is supplied at the top of the log. As you will note, a darkened circle is used to indicate the time when you first get into bed. Even if you have no intention of sleeping just then, but instead are reading a book, having sex, or watching TV, you should still indicate that you are physically in bed by positioning the darkened circle ahead of such activity. This circle should be the last mark you record before morning. *Do not log your sleep and awakenings across the night by consulting a clock. This effort to increase precision will only lead you to become more aware of time passing, and very likely make it harder for you to sleep.*

In the morning, just make your best guess as to when sleep and wakefulness occurred. Use a horizontal line to indicate sleep, interrupted by gaps to indicate wakefulness, as in the example. Indicate the time you actually get out of bed with an open circle. At this juncture, you should also fill in the morning's date, and provide a guess as to how long it took you to fall asleep, once you were actually ready, and estimate how much sleep you accumulated across the night. (We are well aware that many people with insomnia climb into bed with a book or with the TV on to fall asleep. They just let the book drop from their hand if they get lucky and either have the TV set on a timer or else let it rattle on all night. If this describes your preferred approach, simply count the entire interval from the time you got into bed when estimating the time it took you to fall asleep.)

The next evening, as you are darkening a circle on the line below to indicate that you are getting into bed, complete the previous day's log entry by rating your average fatigue level across the day. Use a ten-point scale, with one indicating minimal fatigue—a glorious, high-energy day from start to finish—and ten indicating a day when you could barely function because of overwhelming fatigue.

For example, the insomniac whose interrupted sleep is depicted atop our log got into bed around 12:30 A.M., having taken an antihistamine an hour earlier. Finally falling asleep around 2:15 A.M., she awoke shortly after 5 A.M. and stayed awake for about half an hour. Our diarist accumulated an additional half hour of sleep, beginning shortly before 6 A.M. and then was awake for another hour before rising. It is at this point that she actually filled out the nighttime portion of the log. She first drew an open circle to indicate that she was out of bed. Then she supplied the morning's date, an estimate of how long it took her to first fall asleep, and an estimate of the total amount of sleep accumulated.

The following evening, as our log keeper filled in a darkened circle on the next line to signal getting into bed, she charted events occurring during the day just past that were pertinent to sleep, such as the consumption of caffeinated beverages (using the letter "c") and the occurrence of a half-hour nap around 3:30 P.M. Finally, she rated her average fatigue level during that day, using the ten-point scale just described.

You should feel free to supplement the log with other symbols and notations that may be relevant to your situation. If you consume alcoholic beverages or smoke, you should track this usage. Women who suspect that their sleep difficulties correlate with their menstrual cycles should indicate the phases of that cycle along with their sleep data. If you have wondered how much of an impact seasonal allergies have on your sleep, you may wish to track pollen counts on your log. Make a bunch of fresh copies, because you will be keeping Sleep Logs regularly for the next several weeks—and perhaps intermittently in the coming months as well.

DID YOU LOG A TYPICAL WEEK?

After you have filled out your Sleep Log for one week, you should be ready to determine the basic attributes of your sleep pattern. Understanding this pattern will not only enable us to boost your sleep drive, it will also help in implementing the subsequent steps of your treatment program. However, if after completing your log you realize that it did not capture a representative week, you may need to extend your log keeping for another week or two to get a good sense of your "typical" sleep pattern.

The degree to which your sleep quality varies from week to week could be providing clues about the importance of external factors such as environmental stressors or, for women, internal fluctuations in hormone levels across the menstrual cycle. If your sleep is consistently terrible, one log will indeed look much like another, and it would be safe to assume that changes in hormone levels, job tension, room temperature, garbage pickup, and other potential disruptors are not having much effect. Paradoxically, a similar consistency would result if your sleep is truly haphazard, a different story every night. After all, one sample of chaos looks pretty much like another.

If, on the other hand, your sleep problem is reactive to life events or episodic, you might capture it on one log but not on another. For example, one log might contain a "crunch period" at work. The other might represent a more typical work week. One log might reflect late vigils held as you waited for your teenager to arrive home safely each night during a college break. On the other log, your child might be back at school, at least out of sight if not out of mind. It's likely that you've always had some notion of how closely linked your sleep disturbance is to life events, but now you are finally starting to gather some hard data to back up or refute your suspicions.

FIND YOUR AVERAGE BEDTIME AND AVERAGE RISING TIME

After you have captured a typical week on your Sleep Log, estimate your average bedtime and your average rising time. With a graphic log, this is fairly easy to do. Take a look at the log reproduced here. For simplicity's sake, we've left off everything from the log except the circles indicating bedtime and rising time. At this point, we are not yet adding up your sleep or taking time you spent out of bed into account. Notice that the filled-in circles indicating the week's bedtimes make a sort of cloud. (That is, unless you have taken our sleep hygiene recommendations very much to heart and are getting into bed at exactly the same time every night, in which case they will line up like ducks in a row!) The open circles indicating the times you got out of bed will make another cloud on the other side of the log, something like this:

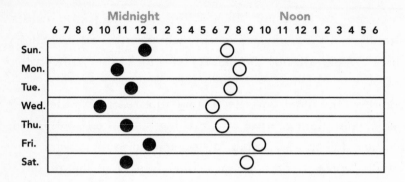

To estimate your average bedtime and rising time for the week, simply divide the clouds in half, as best you can, with a vertical arrow. There should be about as many circles on one side of your arrow as the other. However, if some circles are especially far away from the others (as can happen if you oversleep on weekends!), these may balance out a greater number of circles that end up closer to your dividing arrow, as on the morning side of the following example:

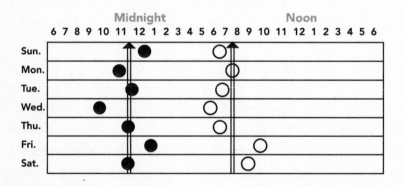

The arrows will point to your average bedtimes—in the case of our example, about 11:15 P.M. and 7:45 A.M. Using your average bedtime and rising time, estimate the average amount of time you spent in bed at night across the week. In our example, this works out to about eight and a half hours. (To arrive at this sum, we added ¾ hours obtained before midnight—that is, from 11:15 P.M. to midnight—to 7 and ¾ hours obtained afterward—that is, from midnight to 7:45 A.M.)

FIND YOUR AVERAGE SLEEP TIME AND AVERAGE WAKE TIME

Your next task is to estimate the average amount of sleep you obtained each night, as well as the average amount of time you spent awake. You have already estimated your total sleep time each night as part of your log-keeping duties. Add up this column for the week, and divide by seven. In our example, this works out to 5.5 hours:

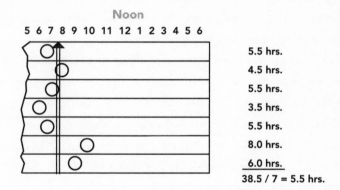

Now, it's a simple matter to calculate the average amount of time you spent awake each night. Just subtract your average total sleep time from the average amount of time you spent in bed. In our example, this calculation would be

8.5 hrs. (avg. time in bed)–5.5 hrs. (avg. sleep time) = 3.0 hrs. (avg. wake time)

CALCULATE YOUR TARGET TIME IN BED

Subtract *half* the average amount of time spent awake on your baseline log from your average bedtime. This will yield the amount of time you should spend in bed during the coming week so as to boost your Sleep Drive and best prime your body for sleep. Following through with our example:

> 8.5 hrs. (avg. time in bed)–1.5 hrs. (½ avg. wake time) = 7.0 hrs. (time in bed)

You should allow yourself seven hours in bed each night. These should be the same seven hours each night to generate a robust wave of sleep. The next step is to determine which seven hours would be best for you. This question will be addressed shortly, after we discuss another way to boost your Sleep Drive.

Note that if you hardly log any sleep at all during your baseline week—say, just one or two hours per night—your assigned time in bed could be very low. To take an extreme example, suppose you average seven hours in bed but believe you sleep only one hour on average, with the other six hours spent awake. This dire situation would yield an assigned bedtime of just four hours in bed per night if no modification were introduced:

> 7 hrs. (avg. time in bed) – 3 hrs. (½ avg. wake time) = 4 hrs. (time in bed)

You need a certain amount of time in bed in which to rest, even if you are not sleeping. For now, we will limit bedtime restriction to six hours. That is, if your calculation yields an assigned bedtime of less than six hours, you should still allow yourself a full six hours in bed. If this moderate restriction of bedtime still produces such undue sleepiness as to interfere with your safely driving a motor vehicle or functioning at work, you should immediately add back some time in bed. Bedtime restriction for you may need to be accomplished in increments of fifteen or thirty minutes, given your apparent sensitivity to sleep loss.

RAISE YOUR BODY TEMPERATURE

Strenuous exercise positioned about four to six hours before bedtime will also boost your Sleep Drive and enhance your prospects for deeper sleep. This effect is not due to muscular fatigue, but rather to the elevation in body temperature (including brain temperature) that accompanies physical exertion. One of the many consequences of sleeping is that it lowers our temperature. When the temperature of the brain is elevated by exercise, it leads to increased amounts of Slow Wave Sleep during the next sleep cycle, apparently as a compensatory cooling effect. The effect appears to be more pronounced in those who are already in very good physical condition.

While strenuous exercise raises temperature, it is also stimulating. You've probably noticed how you can be extremely tired after a vigorous athletic workout but nowhere near the verge of sleep. Just as exercise imposes an artificial "spike" atop the circadian temperature cycle, it also triggers a spurt of arousal. For this reason, it's usually best not to exercise too close to your bedtime. An interval of at least four hours is generally necessary to allow your body to wind down from peak activity.

For the less physically inclined, a similar benefit can be obtained by passively heating the body. It has been found that taking a hot bath about three hours before bedtime can deepen NREM sleep. Researchers used extended immersions to demonstrate the effect; we have obtained good clinical results with a forty-five-minute bath. The water temperature must be quite hot to achieve this effect. Whereas most people will draw a bath of about 90 degrees Fahrenheit, the bath temperature required to enhance sleep is about 103 to 105 degrees. You must be careful here—scalding can occur at temperatures of about 120 degrees Fahrenheit. A number of medical risks are associated with very hot soaks, apart from scalding. This treatment is never appropriate for young children. Others should consult their physicians before beginning such a regimen.

The notion of taking a hot bath three hours before bedtime may

BOOST YOUR SLEEP DRIVE

The **Sleep Drive** is the engine propelling your sleep. You can take steps to increase its power:

- Reduce your time in bed by half the time you typically spend awake each night. (For now, be sure you spend at least six hours in bed.) Within a week or two, you should be falling asleep more quickly. You may get a little less sleep overall, but you will also spend a lot less time tossing and turning.
- Exercise four to six hours before bedtime. Strenuous activity raises your body (and brain) temperature. When the brain's temperature is elevated, it responds with deeper sleep.
- If you are not feeling up to exercising, you can take a hot bath (103 degrees F) for 30 to 45 minutes about three hours before bedtime.

strike you as odd. Conventional wisdom holds that the time to take a bath for the purpose of inducing sleep is just before you get into bed. The discrepancy can be explained if one keeps in mind that many factors interact to promote or interfere with sleep. Some people are primarily inhibited from falling asleep by excessive muscular tension. Their muscles clench and tighten all day long so they are "wound like a spring" by the time they get into bed. For these tense individuals, a conventional bedtime bath may well do more overall good than harm. Others will do better by creating a temperature peak, whether through exercise or soaking in the early evening. This divergence underscores the need to systematically assess the effects of any intervention you make when countering insomnia. Paradoxical results can appear to be more the rule than the exception when dealing with something as slippery as sleep.

Choose the Right Time for Bed

You have just determined how much bedtime you should allow yourself to boost your Sleep Drive. When is it best for you to spend those hours in bed? The short answer to this question is that you should be in bed during those hours when you are most likely to sleep. We will return to your Sleep Log, this time considering the blocks of sleep you charted across the week, to determine those hours. The sleep depicted on your log will probably resemble one of the following three patterns.

1. YOU HAVE DIFFICULTY FALLING ASLEEP

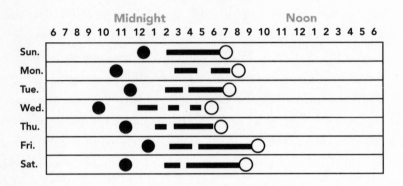

If your sleep tends to follow this pattern, restrict your time in bed by *moving your bedtime later.* Returning to our earlier example, if your average bedtime on the baseline log was 11:15 P.M. and your average rising time was 7:45 A.M., move your bedtime 1.5 hours later, so your new bedtime would be **12:45 A.M.** while your rising time would remain at **7:45 A.M.** This would yield your seven hours in bed.

2. YOU HAVE DIFFICULTY STAYING ASLEEP

Perhaps you have become accustomed to getting out of bed during the early morning hours to surf the Internet, watch television or get started on housework.

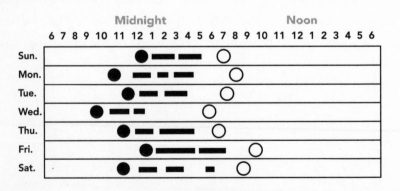

If your sleep tends to follow this pattern, restrict your time in bed by *moving your rising time earlier*. Returning to our example, your bedtime would remain **11:15** P.M., but your new rising time would be **6:15** A.M., again yielding seven hours in bed.

3. YOUR SLEEP IS BROKEN THROUGHOUT THE NIGHT

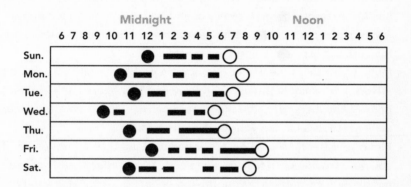

If your sleep resembles this pattern, you should restrict your bedtime by cutting half the excess bedtime from each end of the night, *moving your bedtime later and your rising time earlier*. Returning yet again to our example, you would move your bedtime 45 minutes later, to **12 midnight** and your rising time 45 minutes earlier, to **7** A.M.

Once you have determined the right time to be in bed, you should log at least one week on your new schedule.

CHOOSE THE RIGHT TIME FOR BED

The best sleep results when pent-up **Sleep Drive** is unleashed at the right time—that is, when the **Alerting Force** is waning.

- Move your bedtime later if your main problem is difficulty falling asleep. Cut half the time you usually spend awake out of your schedule. For example, if you typically spend two hours awake in bed, primarily at the start of the night, set your new bedtime one hour later than usual. Keep your rising time constant.
- Move your rising time earlier if your main problem is difficulty staying asleep. For example, if you typically spend two hours awake in bed, primarily at the end of the night, set your new rising time one hour earlier than usual. Keep your bedtime constant.
- Move your bedtime a little later and your rising time a little earlier if you have trouble both falling asleep and staying asleep, or if you cannot discern any pattern in your broken sleep. For example, if you typically spend two hours awake in bed scattered throughout the night, set your new bedtime one-half hour later and your new rising time one-half hour earlier than usual.

Differentiate Your Therapy

These simple changes will soon be introducing some regularity into your sleep experience. It's clear that you can't have a great night of sleep on this shortened bedtime routine; there's not enough time. However, you will begin to see that you don't have many terrible nights either. Your sleep will become more predictable, as homeostatic mechanisms begin to boost your Sleep Drive and as you position your bedtime at the circadian phase when you are most likely to catch a wave of sleep. For some of you, our Preliminary Treatment will suffice to right your sleep and set it on a reliable course. For those of you whose sleep is still feeling wobbly, we are now ready to apply treatments specifically matched to your particular type of insomnia.

These treatments are presented in the next three chapters. If you identified yourself as someone who has a hard time getting to sleep and who sleeps best in the morning, you should proceed to Chapter 6 when you have finished reading this chapter. If you don't have much problem falling asleep but tend to awaken too early and are unable to resume your slumbers, you should skip to Chapter 7. Finally, if your sleep is broken into short fragments, if you experience awakenings in the middle of the night, or if you cannot discern a pattern to your sleep at all, Chapter 8 is where your next steps may be found.

Ease Your Mind

We have emphasized throughout this book that good sleep flows from a cooperative agreement between the body and the mind. The experience of chronic insomnia threatens both parties to this pact: the body's circadian system loses its fine tuning and instead begins to clunk along like an engine that is misfiring. The mind, meanwhile, loses its confidence that sleep will occur automatically and instead starts to obsessively micromanage the process. When trying to restore sleep to reliable functioning, we first work on physiological misalignment, in part because we can thereby improve sleep at least a little, even while anxiety runs unchecked. Demonstration of this improvement in turn should help allay the mind's doubt that sleep will ever return.

Eventually, however, we will need to soothe your mind directly. There are a number of ways to accomplish this goal. We have already begun the process by asking you to question attitudes and beliefs that may be getting in the way of your sleeping well. Relaxation Training and Guided Imagery are also very useful when it comes to preparing the mind for sleep.

RELAXATION TRAINING

The aim of Relaxation Training is to promote calm through body awareness. Often we are not fully aware of the tension we carry within ourselves, even though it may manifest itself through shallow or forced breathing, clenched muscles, an elevated heart rate, or other physical signs. By learning to recognize these changes, and especially by distinguishing between varying levels of tension so we can aim for a progressively quieter physical state, we buffer the body against stress, which in turn helps to calm the mind.

GUIDED IMAGERY

We humans like to think—if unable to sleep at two in the morning, we are unlikely to keep our minds blank. Instead, we are prone to dwelling on jingles, shopping lists, dilemmas, deadlines, or most ominously, the fact that we are not sleeping. This stream of information is likely to keep us awake even longer. Fortunately, our minds are also open to suggestion regarding things to think about. Guided Imagery makes therapeutic use of the truth that we cannot consciously entertain more than one image in our minds at a time. The treatment gently pushes distressing thoughts to the back of the queue, out of mind, while it substitutes a more tranquil image up front.

Before we even climb into bed we can prepare a restful scene, such as a white sandy beach with turquoise water rippling and golden palm trees swaying. As we repeatedly visit this refuge by day or evening, we can fill in additional details so it will be that much more convincing by night. We can develop a mental itinerary that whisks us to a sun-washed seaside villa, down a short path to the left, under a generous red umbrella, and onto a cushioned lounge chair positioned to catch the breeze. This route should become so familiar, so well-trodden, that it practically pulls you along when you embark upon it in bed.

Relaxation Training and Guided Imagery are employed by many cognitive-behavioral therapists—it is not necessary to find a sleep specialist to receive instruction in these techniques. These methods are also the subjects of many helpful books and tapes. In addition, we will be providing specific examples of how to use Relaxation Training and Guided Imagery to ease your mind in the last chapter. For now, you should be aware that these techniques can be of great benefit to you regardless of the type of insomnia you are struggling with. They will complement rather than interfere with the more specific treatments you will soon be following.

CHAPTER SIX

Answers for Difficulty Falling Asleep

Difficulty falling asleep is a problem of traversing the boundary between two states. Just as when one country, in clamping down on its border, creates congestion, delays, and flaring tempers on its neighbor's side of the crossing, when we have difficulty entering sleep, anxiety backs up into our waking hours. We begin to anticipate the predicament we will be facing several hours later. This anxiety in turn interferes with the process of gradually winding down that should precede the descent into sleep. We also grow to mistrust our bedrooms and our beds and can feel ourselves tightening up inside as we drag ourselves from living or family rooms (places that put few demands upon us) to enter the dreaded bedchamber. It's no surprise, therefore, that many people with this type of insomnia end up falling asleep more readily on couches and in recliners, where the stakes are low. Usually this slumber is short lived, and it renders the prospects of returning to sleep in bed even less likely.

As we address the various manifestations of difficulty falling asleep in this chapter, you'll notice that many of the interventions we suggest actually take place during waking hours, either before or after sleep. We may be making changes to your bedtime schedule, to your pattern of light exposure, to the way you deal with problems in the evening, or to other aspects of your daily life. This is not by accident: *how easily you will make the transition into sleep is in large part decided outside of bed*. We have many strategies to ease you across this threshold, even if lately it has been taking you several hours. We will start, however, by tackling some less-drastic problems.

Problem: Sunday Night Insomnia

Take a look at your original Sleep Log. Focusing first on variation within the week itself, do you have the classic "Sunday Night Insomnia" pattern?

Date	Morning's Time to Fall Asleep	Amount of Sleep	Fatigue Rating 1 Lo–10 Hi
Mo 12/10	120 min.	5 1/2 hrs	2
Tu 12/11	70 min.	6 hrs	6
We 12/12	35 min.	6 1/2 hrs	7
Th 12/13	25 min.	7 1/2 hrs	6
Fr 12/14	5 min.	7 1/2 hrs	4
Sat 12/15	5 min.	7 1/2 hrs + 1/4 hrs	3
Sun 12/16	0 min.	8 1/4 hrs	2

The apprehension that builds as the start of the work or school week approaches can certainly lead to sleeplessness, especially in those who are already half-expecting poor sleep anyway and wondering how they will be able to function the following day. Other factors potentially contributing to this pattern are oversleeping on Saturday and Sunday mornings, which begins to delay the circadian propensity for sleep, and weekend napping, which uses up some of the drive for sleep prematurely, before Sunday night even arrives.

ANSWER: LIMIT WEEKEND OVERSLEEPING

If your pattern resembles the one shown in the preceding example, it's time to make a pact with yourself about the amount of weekend oversleeping you will allow. We have found that the Sleep Hygiene rule about getting up at the same time on workdays and weekends is very difficult for most people to adhere to, especially if they tend to stay up later on weekend nights. Rather than proclaiming good intentions, setting an early alarm, and then sleeping through it, it's better to acknowledge that you need to oversleep at least a little for the morning to feel like a weekend. However, you should control the amount of extra time you allow yourself in bed.

Spending one extra hour in bed on weekends may not sound like much, but after a few weeks, you will come to appreciate the difference. The catch here is that even if you stay out very late on Friday night, finally collapsing into bed three hours after your usual bedtime, you *still* get only one extra hour in bed. You will have to trade off some sleep against your socializing. It's a misconception that you need to stay at home in the evening if you have trouble falling asleep. You can still go out at night; however, you may find that you don't want to stay out quite so late on weekend nights, if you are really serious about addressing this insomnia pattern.

We will soon be considering the special problems facing adolescents and young adults with regard to late-night sleep patterns. For now, suffice it to say that weekend oversleeping of four or five hours, relative to the very early weekday rising time young people need to make a school bus, is not at all uncommon. In these cases, weekend oversleeping needs to be addressed as part of a more comprehensive treatment approach. It may make sense to compromise at least initially on a weekend rising time two or three hours later than the weekday time.

Problem: It Usually Takes an Hour to Fall Asleep

In consulting your Sleep Log, observe how long, on average, it takes you to fall asleep after you turn out the lights. Does your pattern look something like this?

	Morning's Date	Time to Fall Asleep	Amount of Sleep	Fatigue Rating 1 Lo–10 Hi
	Mo 6/3	60 min.	7 1/2 hrs	3
	Tu 6/4	70 min.	7 3/4 hrs	5
	We 6/5	60 min.	7 1/4 hrs	5
	Th 6/6	60 min.	6 hrs	7
	Fr 6/7	60 min.	6 3/4 hrs	6
	Sat 6/8	55 min.	8 hrs	6
	Sun 6/9	50 min.	8 1/2 hrs	4

ANSWER: MAINTAIN A "BUFFER PERIOD"

If it often takes you about sixty minutes to fall asleep across the entire week (not just on weekends as discussed earlier), you may be winding down after you get into bed, rather than beforehand. This kind of problem can often be resolved by making sure you have an adequate "buffer period" between the end of physically demanding, emotionally stimulating, or anxiety provoking evening activities (e.g., volleyball practice, drawn-out phone calls, paying bills) and the start of bedtime. During this buffer period, your goal is to be pleasantly diverted but not overly concerned with what you are doing. Reading magazine articles makes for an effective buffer period activity, because such articles are usually written in a direct, easy-to-digest style, and are short enough to finish in a sitting. Listening to music, quiet conversation, or watching sitcoms (while avoiding the nightly news!) can work as well. You will know that you have chosen an appropriate buffer activity if you are engaged enough to be unaware of the passage of time and still distracted from any issues of real personal significance.

Late evening is often the time couples finally find the opportunity to deal with pressing concerns. The chores are finished. If young children are in the home, they are in bed. Mutual procrastination has allowed thorny problems to proliferate. Even though it seems you have no choice but to tackle these problems before bedtime, resist the urge to do so. Your patience will likely be worn thin by then, and the heated arguments that ensue will surely be resonating in your head for hours, crowding out any opportunity for sweet dreams. Instead, make an appointment with your partner to address difficult issues the following day, in an earlier timeslot. Learn to preserve the hours before bedtime as a conflict-free time zone.

We previously employed the metaphor of piloting a plane toward landing to illustrate how you should prepare yourself for sleep. Just as a pilot calculates a rate of descent based on current altitude and the distance remaining to the airport, you must take stock of your level of arousal in relation to how long it is until bedtime. It does no good in either instance to be making too steep a descent. You don't want to be on the verge of sleep at 8:30 P.M., dozing or fending off sleep for hours, only to have trouble falling asleep when it really counts. At the same time, you want to be ready to touch down, whether on a runway or in the comfort of your bed, when the time is right.

So make a habit of checking your level of arousal as the evening progresses, and make corrections as you enter your "final approach." If you find yourself bleary-eyed in the recliner early in the evening, get up and fold some clothes or straighten up your desk. Do not attempt anything too strenuous—just find enough activity to avoid falling asleep. On the other hand, if your self-check turns up evidence of hyperarousal, be sure you use your remaining hours of wakefulness to fashion a calmer mind-set, and a more relaxed bodily state, before you turn out the light.

ANSWER: GAUGE YOUR READINESS FOR SLEEP

We have devised and tested a strategy to gauge your readiness for sleep in the evening. To employ this strategy, briefly plumb the level of your sleepiness on the hour: turn off all audio and visual distractions, and find a quiet, comfortable place in which to either lie down or recline. Close your eyes, and be still for about one minute. Rate your sleepiness/readiness for sleep on a scale from 1 (not at all sleepy) to 10 (very sleepy). Write down your rating, and repeat this procedure each hour until your bedtime. This process will prepare you for sleep, because you will learn to recognize your personal "rate of descent." You may notice, for example, that sleepiness for you is not very apparent until right before bedtime. Or you may be able to detect gradually increasing sleepiness throughout the evening.

If on a given night something is acting to deflect you from your typical pattern so you do not sense a readiness for sleep, you may do well to push your bedtime back a bit. (Be careful about bedtime adjustments in the opposite direction, however. If you go to bed earlier than usual, even if you're feeling sleepy, this can lead to difficulty falling or staying asleep. In the case of prematurely appearing sleepiness, you may want to gently increase your level of evening activity as described earlier.)

GAUGE YOUR SLEEPINESS IN THE EVENING

Each hour, find a quiet, comfortable place in which to either lie down or recline. Close your eyes, and be still for about one minute.

Rate your sleepiness/readiness for sleep on a scale from 1 (not at all sleep/not ready to sleep) to 10 (very sleepy/ready for sleep).

Your pattern of sleepiness in the evening will help you prepare for sleep and know when to adjust your activity level or your bedtime.

ANSWER: SET ASIDE "WORRY TIME"

Sitting yourself down in a comfortable chair and facing your worries head on, before your buffer period begins, will help you find your way to sleep more quickly when you do climb into bed. We illustrated in a previous chapter just how varied and idiosyncratic the range of thoughts and worries impinging upon sleep can be. Preset questionnaires can hardly do justice to this diversity. Therefore, you should keep a journal of the thoughts floating around in your mind during the evening to get a better sense of your personal concerns. Divide each page of the journal with a vertical line down the middle. Then relax in a chair for about twenty minutes, listing your concerns on the left half of the page as they occur to you. You will probably find that some of the worries on which your mind is dwelling before sleep are as prosaic as unpaid bills or work deadlines, while other concerns are surprising or even mystifying.

We are not asking you to dredge up these worries merely to fill a notebook. Your assignment does not end until you have come to at least a temporary resolution regarding any troubling issues. Don't worry about finding an optimal solution. You do not have to come up with enough funds hidden under the mattress to pay the bills. You do not have to actually complete the presentation you are slotted to give at the office next week. All you have to do is solve the problem for the night to get yourself off the hook. This might mean convincing yourself that you have a plan to accomplish your goal, that the problem is not really that big after all, or that if necessary, you have some fallback options. List your temporary solutions on the right side of the journal page, across from the problems for which they provide a fix.

The remedies you come up with during this evening ritual may appear flimsy—and would appear even more so by the light of day! *How are such obviously contrived answers going to allow me to sleep?* you may be thinking. Not to worry. Your mind at night is not the most rigorous thinker. Just as it has a tendency to catastrophize while you lay in bed, exaggerating the shadow cast by problems, it can also be persuaded to buttress your rickety solutions. A part of you does want to sleep, after all, and this part will be desperate for any material it can employ in rebuttal when confronted with a challenge.

In fact, the simple act of writing down your worries will have a salutary effect. Have you ever noticed how a fear of forgetting to do something important can set off a cyclone of obsessive "remembering"? Suppose you must deposit a check before the bank closes but are stuck at work. Every two minutes, it seems, you remind yourself to run this errand on your lunch break. You finally break this cycle by sticking a note to yourself on your computer screen, because only then do you feel assured that you will not forget.

Although it may seem unlikely that you are worried about forgetting all the flotsam drifting around in your head at night, on some level, that anxiety is exactly what is keeping it afloat. Simply by being able to say to yourself, *Yes, I know all about you—you are listed on page 3. I've got a fix in mind, and I'll see you in the morning* can allow your mind to stand down for the night.

ANSWER: FOLLOW STIMULUS CONTROL INSTRUCTIONS

If you have prepared yourself for sleep as described earlier but still find yourself awake for an hour after you get into bed, it is time for you to apply Stimulus Control Instructions. This deceptively straightforward treatment, developed by Richard Bootzin, applies well-established learning principles to repeatedly foster the experience of falling asleep soon after you climb into bed. This may be just the experience you need to break the maladaptive association that has likely been forged between your bed and sleeplessness. The treatment limits the amount of time you spend in bed awake (whether actually trying to fall asleep or engaged in such activities as reading, eating, and television viewing) and has you return to bed only when you are ready to fall asleep.

We apply Stimulus Control Instructions as follows:

1. If you are not asleep within about twenty minutes, *get out of bed.*

2. Don't get back into bed until you are sleepy or feel you can fall asleep.

3. Once in bed, repeat #1.

4. Do not use the bed for anything besides sleep and sex.

5. Wake up at the same time every weekday. (You can sleep one hour later on weekends.)

6. Don't nap.

You will be getting out of bed quite often at the start of treatment. So prepare yourself with light reading such as magazines and newspapers you can peruse in a sitting. Do not try to complete overdue tax forms or tackle household chores; do not dive into engrossing novels or begin watching the first installment of some nine-hour video saga. These kinds of activities are too stimulating—they can stoke alertness, prolonging what might have otherwise been a short prep for sleep into half a night of entertainment or work.

Many patients find that it can take up to an hour before they feel sleepy enough to get back into bed. So for a few weeks, you will likely lose even more sleep than usual. Try not to worry about this. Applying Stimulus Control Instructions will result in your falling to sleep more rapidly when you do allow yourself back into bed. For the moment, this is more important than the lost sleep, because you need to prove to yourself that you can in fact fall asleep rapidly. During the day, however, you should expect some increased fatigue and irritability. With time, you will start getting to sleep more rapidly, and any residual fatigue will be less troublesome.

ANSWER: USE MELATONIN TO INDUCE SLEEP

Melatonin is a hormone produced by the pineal gland, which is located at the base of the brain. Melatonin is currently receiving intense scrutiny from both sleep researchers and clinicians because it first appears in twilight and continues to be released only in the dark. When morning light enters the eye, melatonin levels quickly drop. Therefore, melatonin not only displays a circadian rhythm but also acts as the body's link to the external light/dark cycle.

Supplemental melatonin in doses as low as 0.3 milligram induces sleepiness and helps individuals fall asleep faster—two features particularly useful in addressing the problem of difficulty falling asleep that we are considering here. It is available from health food and vitamin stores without a prescription, and it is typically used in doses ranging from a fraction of 1 milligram to about 10 milligrams.

The sleep-inducing effect of melatonin is relatively mild when compared to that of prescription sleeping pills. Similarly, its ability to alter biological rhythms is less potent than that of timed exposure to bright light, a treatment we will be considering shortly. Its effectiveness appears to result from a combination of its mild hypnotic effect and its ability to shift circadian rhythms. It acts on *both* the Sleep Drive and the Alerting Force. Because of these unique properties, melatonin is best taken about three to four hours before bedtime rather than just before getting into bed. As we write, a new prescription medication that works in the brain in a manner similar to melatonin is being introduced. Initial trials have shown that this medication is superior to melatonin in promoting rapid sleep onset.

Melatonin is useful in hastening sleep onset both when sleep is typically delayed by one hour, as we have been discussing, and when sleep is delayed by several hours—a problem we will be considering in the next section.

It has been shown to help induce naps, a strategy often advised for shift workers. Melatonin is also capable of synchronizing the circadian rhythms of totally blind individuals, who otherwise often have difficulty aligning their sleep schedules to meet work or school obligations. However, melatonin does not appear to be as useful in keeping people sleeping through the night. This may be due to the fact that it is already being secreted during dark hours, so any effects of an extra dose are masked. By contrast, when taken during the day or early evening, supplemental melatonin is not competing with the naturally occurring hormone.

Problem: It Usually Takes Several Hours to Fall Asleep

If your Sleep Log shows that it routinely takes you two, three, or more hours to fall asleep at the start of the night, while you typically oversleep late into the morning (causing significant problems at work or at school), it's probable that you have a distinct circadian rhythm disorder known as delayed sleep phase disorder. There is likely a physiologically based mismatch between the time you (or your boss, or your parents) *think* you should fall asleep and the time your body is actually *ready* to sleep. As we discussed in Chapter 3, a delayed sleep phase is often based at least in part on individual differences in the workings of an internal circadian pacemaker. A young patient of ours named Vijay typified this clinical picture. Here is the Sleep Log he filled out prior to our first meeting:

Morning's Date	Time to Fall Asleep	Amount of Sleep	Fatigue Rating 1 Lo–10 Hi
Mo 12/10	110 min.	4 1/2 hrs	5
Tu 12/11	80 min.	4 hrs	7
We 12/12	120 min.	5 hrs	7
Th 12/13	210 min.	6 hrs + 1 1/2 hrs	9
Fr 12/14	130 min.	8 1/2 hrs	7
Sat 12/15	5 min.	11 hrs	5
Sun 12/16	0 min.	9 1/2 hrs	2

Vijay, a fifteen-year-old high school student on academic probation, trailed his mother into the consultation room. He was a bright student who was used to squeaking through with As in his classes despite frequent absence and tardiness. His mother reported that he had always liked to stay up at night, even in early childhood. However, in the last year, Vijay's sleep problem had gotten out of hand. He had missed his first-period biology class thirty-five times last semester because she couldn't get him out of bed.

Vijay would go to bed shortly after midnight on school nights, but he would end up listening to music or playing computer games until well past 2 A.M., even though his alarm was set for 5:45 A.M. His mother needed close to an hour to practically pull him out of the bed, giving Vijay just fifteen minutes to eat, dress, and run two blocks to the bus stop. Vijay would resume sleeping immediately on the bus, and continue dozing throughout his morning classes. Staying awake in the afternoon was less of a problem, and he finally felt fully alert after dinner.

A few nights of just four or five hours sleep would eventually catch up with Vijay, and by Wednesday or Thursday, he was virtually impossible to rouse in the morning. Vijay's mother would give up, letting her son sleep past noon. He followed a similar late pattern on weekends, not even getting into bed until two or three in the morning and sleeping half the day away, ready to repeat the cycle in the coming week.

If your Sleep Log resembles Vijay's, you need to advance the timing of your sleep. As you have no doubt learned, this involves more than simply getting into bed earlier. You have likely been getting that advice for years, and it probably just leads to extra hours spent tossing and turning before you finally fall asleep. Several available treatments stand a better chance of success.

ANSWER: CHRONOTHERAPY

The earliest treatment for delayed sleep phase disorder, proposed just a few years after the syndrome was described, makes use of the fact that it is easier for almost everyone (and especially night owls) to sleep soundly after staying awake an extra few hours, compared to the difficulty of sleeping well when going to bed earlier than usual. This treatment, named *Chronotherapy*, brings patients around to earlier bedtimes by progressively shifting their sleep *later* "around the clock." The process is analogous to traveling westward around the world—as you near the end of your global circuit, you will find yourself due *east* of where you first started out.

Suppose your sleep pattern closely matches Vijay's. Examination of your logs shows that you don't usually fall asleep until around 3 A.M., regardless of when you get into bed. You may want to institute Chronotherapy to shift your sleep phase to earlier hours. To administer this treatment, you may have to take a temporary leave from work or school or else wait for a vacation break, as Chronotherapy requires a week or so when you do not have to meet your typical daily obligations.

First, regulate your bedtime to a 3 A.M. to 10 A.M. schedule for four nights. Note that this schedule yields seven hours in bed, even though you would probably prefer to have eight or more. It's important to introduce a mild amount of bedtime restriction to keep sleep consolidated during the process of shifting your sleep phase. Compared with the four to five hours of sleep you are probably accumulating on weekdays as you wrench yourself out of bed in the morning, the slight restriction of bedtime will probably not incur any additional sleep loss.

Following this short period of bedtime stabilization, begin a series of progressive three-hour delays in your bedtime. On the first night, stay up until 6 A.M. and set your alarm for 1 P.M. While these hours might strike some readers as outlandish, in fact they likely represent a typical "late night" for you. However, on the following night, you should wait until 9 A.M. before going to bed, rising at 4 P.M. Here's where things may get a bit more difficult. For the first time in perhaps a very long while, you will actually want to go to sleep earlier than your assigned bedtime. You must resist this urge to turn in, instead keeping yourself active during the early morning hours. Perhaps you might be able to recruit some early risers at home to help you stay awake. After four more phase shifts, your assigned bedtime will arrive at 9 P.M. to 4 A.M. During this sequence of shifts, you will effectively be living on a twenty-seven-hour "day." Your allotted bedtimes across this sequence, including the period of stabilization, would look like this:

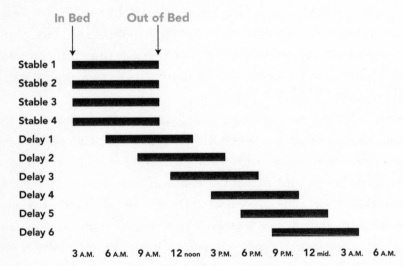

At this point, you should delay your bedtime more gradually while expanding the amount of time you spend in bed slightly. For example, you might spend three nights with an assigned bedtime of 9:30 P.M. to 5 A.M. and then the next three nights with a bedtime of 10 P.M. to 5:30 A.M. before you reach your ultimate goal.

Chronotherapy can be quite effective, introducing rapid change into a situation that may have been intractable for years. It does have its pitfalls, however. Oftentimes, the first phase shifts are easiest to execute, but in the middle of the schedule, you will be keeping very awkward hours, trying to sleep in the afternoon and evening when you were used to seeing friends, making appointments, and running errands. It helps to enlist family and friends in this effort, both to schedule some social interaction at odd hours and to alert them against calling or visiting when you are planning to sleep. Blackout curtains and an answering machine that can silently take your phone calls are also helpful.

Another potential pitfall with Chronotherapy is that it does not provide much opportunity to stabilize your sleep cycle on an early pattern, so it is very easy to zip right past your targeted bedtime back to a late schedule if you do not take precautions. That is why we recommend that you phase shift fairly quickly at first but then slow down to a delay of perhaps one hour and finally half an hour every three days, so as not to overshoot the mark. We also suggest that you "apply the brakes" once you reach your desired bedtime through timed exposure to bright light, as will be described in the next section.

In practice, we recommend that you employ Chronotherapy only if the sun has usually risen by the time you actually fall asleep. Otherwise, we would suggest that you very gradually *advance* the timing of your sleep phase through regulation of bedtimes and carefully timed exposure to bright light.

ANSWER: BRIGHT LIGHT TREATMENT

Sometimes a process can take place so seamlessly as to become transparent—and thereby difficult to see. Such is the case with the regulation of sleep by bright light. We discussed early on that, like most animals, we humans typically display a more or less predictable sleep pattern: most of us are *diurnal*, active by day while sleeping primarily during the night. Some of us emulate *nocturnal* animals, coming to life at sundown while inactive during the day. One might not think to ask how we (let alone the rest of the animal kingdom) know what time it is, and by extension when it is time to sleep. After all, like other animals we have eyes to see—even before the invention of clocks we could always tell whether the sun was up or not! That is true enough, but not the whole story.

Over the past fifty years, a revolution has taken place in our understanding of the intricate way in which our sleep is linked to the rising and setting sun. Paradoxically, this research reestablishes a central role for the sun in our circadian system, just as surely as it once occupied the center of the Copernican universe.

The study of circadian rhythms can be traced back to the French astronomer Jean Jacques de Mairan, who in 1729 demonstrated that the heliotrope, a plant known to raise and open its leaves by day and fold them down at night, would continue its daily and nightly movements even when covered up and isolated from all traces of light. This was the first demonstration of an *endogenous* circadian rhythm, that is, a function regulated by an internal clock rather than by external cues. As we learned in Chapter 3, much of our physiology is regulated by this internal clock. Beginning in the 1960s, researchers began to piece together the story of how the "hands" of this internal clock are set by exposure to light, as well as, to a lesser extent, by other time cues.

Recall from Chapter 2 that the circadian temperature rhythm is a good proxy for the Alerting Force that counters our Sleep Drive each day and night. This temperature rhythm reaches a peak (in those of us who regularly sleep at night) in the early evening, and it has its low point in the very early morning, slightly more than two hours before we typically awaken. Exposure to bright light (which until about a hundred years ago was supplied exclusively by the sun) can shift the timing of our sleep phase, making it easier or more difficult to sleep at a given time of day or night. The direction and magnitude of the shift has been worked out for humans and other animals; it can be predicted by a mathematical function known as a *phase response curve*. It is not imperative that you understand fully the workings of the phase response curve to improve your chances of being met with sleep when you climb into bed. All that is really necessary to remember is this:

If you are exposed to bright light shortly before or during the first two thirds of your habitual sleep period, your sleep phase will tend to shift *later*. If you are exposed to bright light in the last third of your sleep period or shortly thereafter, your sleep phase will tend to shift *earlier*.

Note that if we are exposed to bright light in the middle of the day—the time most of us will have that experience, if we're lucky enough to get outside—such exposure may be healthy and good for our spirits, but it usually will not have much effect on the timing of our sleep.

How much light exposure one needs to trigger such sleep phase shifts is a question that has prompted sophisticated research protocols in recent years. Most people are not aware of the vast difference in intensity between the artificial lights we typically use in our homes and workplaces and the natural light available just outside our doors. What we consider a bright room with ample lighting fixtures supplementing a few windows may register an intensity of about 400 lux on a light meter held at its center. If that same meter were to be carried outdoors at noon on a summer day, it might register 100,000 lux. Even the supposedly pale gray sky of early dawn, with the sun just over the horizon, would yield about 2,500 lux. Our eyes are clearly not the best judges of intensity. That is because they are more geared to judging contrasts than absolute levels.

Initial research on the phase-shifting effects of light tended to employ devices that mimicked pale evening or dawn light—that is, about 2,500 or 10,000 lux—for one or two hours. In our clinical practice, we have obtained good treatment responses by recommending that patients go outdoors at designated times for at least thirty minutes or, if that is impractical, acquire a commercially available lamp or lightbox that provides intensities of about 10,000 lux when positioned about a foot and a half to two feet away.

Unlike tanning lights, these units should emit low levels of ultraviolet light, so as to avoid harm to the skin and eyes despite daily use. In addition to standard bright light devices, light visors are currently available, and glasses with small light-emitting diodes attached to their lenses are being introduced as well. These light sources allow one to soak up sufficient light while moving about, making them more practical for use during the morning rush to prepare for school or work.

More recent research suggests that prolonged (e.g., five or six hours') exposure to light of much lower intensity, similar to levels typically encountered indoors or even lower, can have phase-shifting effects when people usually spend their waking hours in dimly lit rooms. This finding does not substantially alter our recommendations regarding the use of bright light treatment, because brighter light is more effective at producing phase shifts. However, it does make us more vigilant regarding the potential effects of incidental light exposure.

For example, our colleagues Mark Rea, Mariana Figueiro, and John Bullough at the Lighting Research Center of Rensselaer Polytechnic Institute have calculated that peering into a brightly glowing standard-size computer screen positioned twelve inches away for three hours causes about a 25 percent suppression of melatonin—the mechanism, you may recall, by which our circadian rhythms are linked to the light/dark cycle produced by the earth's rotation. In other words, spending hours in front of a computer screen (especially late at night) may alter our circadian rhythms. Those of us with teenagers locked in their bedrooms, noses glued to oversized screens as they instant message into the wee hours, have seen the effects of this firsthand.

Perhaps the most astounding news that has emanated from research into light and the circadian system is the discovery of a new type of receptor in the eye that is directly associated with the circadian clock. These receptors are distinct from the rods and cones that, you may recall from middle school, are responsible for vision. Nestled in the retina, they managed to escape detection by generations of anatomists until a few years ago. They are most sensitive to light of around 480 nanometers (corresponding to the deep blue of the sky) and are, therefore, known as blue-light receptors. These newly discovered receptors work in concert with other photoreceptors in the retina to alert the circadian system to the presence of light. The circadian system as a whole is, therefore, maximally sensitive to light of slightly shorter wavelengths, between 440 to 450 nanometers. Professor Rea and his colleagues coined the term "blue-sky detector" to describe this portal into the circadian system.

This discovery has profound importance for all who are hoping to establish a reliable rhythm of sleep and wakefulness. Carefully timed exposure to light (specifically, to light in that part of the spectrum acting on the blue-sky detecting circadian system) can be of direct benefit to those of you who are contending with a delayed sleep phase, shift work, and many other conditions associated with sleep disturbance.

Setting Up Your Bright-Light Device

If you have any eye problems other than the common types corrected with glasses, you should check with your doctor before using bright-light therapy. More manufacturers are marketing units employing less-intense light tuned to the shorter wavelengths of the spectrum, which may be more appropriate for you. When using a light box, you should follow the manufacturer's recommendations regarding placement. Thirty minutes typically represents a minimum exposure time for effective treatment. You may require forty-five minutes, an hour, or longer. Fortunately, a light box allows the possibility of having breakfast, catching up on the morning's news, or doing some homework while you use it.

You do not have to stare into the light. Many people with a delayed sleep phase are photophobic—the last thing they want to see in the morning is bright light, and some people even get headaches from too intense an exposure. You may need to experiment with placement a foot or so farther away. However, the intensity of light falls off rapidly as its source recedes—doubling the distance, for example, will lower the intensity to just one fourth of its original level—so you will not receive an effective dose of light if the unit is pushed across the room, even though it will continue to look very bright. In addition, it is important that the light source not be placed too much to one side. If the angle between the light box and the direction in which you are looking is too great, the amount of light that actually enters your eyes will be insufficient.

One final caveat: if you have been diagnosed with bipolar disorder, formerly known as manic-depression, you should be aware that bright light therapy may trigger a manic episode. You should consult with your physician before beginning this type of treatment.

Scheduling Your Bright-Light Treatment

Suppose your sleep log demonstrates a pattern matching Vijay's—the time you actually fall asleep is about four hours later than your desired bedtime of about 11 P.M. Before you begin to advance your sleep phase, first regulate your sleep to late, mildly restricted bedtime hours—for example, to between 3 A.M. and 10:30 A.M. Set aside a one-hour "buffer period" before bedtime for reading to give yourself an opportunity to wind down. Log off your computer and turn off your cell phone as well.

You should set at least two alarm clocks or rely on others to be sure you are out of bed at 10:30 A.M., and obtain bright light exposure starting at 11 A.M. (The onset of the light should be two hours before your typical weekend rising time. If, like Vijay, you would consistently sleep to about 1 P.M. when given the chance, we would recommend that your morning light exposure start at 11 A.M.) If you do not have a light box, this means pulling on some clothes and getting outdoors for at least thirty minutes. In the summer months, you can just sit if you would like; in cooler weather, you may have to bundle up and take a walk. If the weather is particularly treacherous, we do not suggest that you go outdoors. Instead, you can garner some benefit from sitting in a sunroom or by an eastern or southern window during your allotted exposure time.

Note that you will likely be late for school or work for a while as you address this problem. In practice, we endeavor to explain this procedure ahead of time to school principals or work supervisors to enlist their support. Oftentimes, after dealing with the problem unsuccessfully for a year or longer, they are quite willing to wait a month or so to get it resolved.

As proposed in our earlier discussion of Sunday Night Insomnia, we suggest that you allow yourself one extra hour in bed on weekends as a reward for getting through the week. As soon as you get out of bed you should obtain at least a full hour of light exposure if you do not have to run off to meet some obligation. After your light treatment, you should explore the possibilities that weekend mornings and early afternoons have to offer. We know that morning always seemed a harsh and barren zone, useless for anything except sleeping, but it does have its charms. You can engage in some favorite outdoor activity, indulge in a hobby, or meet a friend for coffee. Alternatively, you might just want to putter around the house wasting time, because even if you do, you still will have plenty of hours left in your day.

After one week on this schedule, move your "buffer period," bedtime, rising time, and light exposure earlier by one hour, both on weekdays and weekends. Although this doesn't seem like much progress, it is in fact your best route to success. The circadian rhythms supporting your sleep may be able to shift more quickly in a laboratory setting, but in the real world, you are also pushing up against all the engrained patterns and preferences that have accrued during your years as a night owl: your favorite late-night TV shows, your urge to call friends for midnight chats, your best hours of clear-headed thinking when the house is quiet. You will need some time to get used to the concept of midnight being "late." Within a few weeks, you will be able to show up noticeably earlier to work or to school. You should do so, rather than waiting until you are fully phase shifted before appearing at the desired start time.

We have set forth a particularly protracted schedule of phase advancement here, one which in our clinical experience maximizes the likelihood of success for the most difficult cases. However, we are aware that some people are more able to advance their sleep phase on a physiological basis, while others may be more motivated to do so by the combination of inducements and punishments they face. If you find that your first one or two phase shifts have gone off without a hitch, you may be able to accelerate the schedule. You can try shifting an hour every three or four days to get close to your targeted sleep schedule more quickly.

However, as recommended in our discussion of Chronotherapy, we suggest that you then reduce the extent of your shifts as you approach your desired target, perhaps moving your bedtime earlier by thirty minutes at each step. You are in little danger here of overshooting the mark and falling asleep too early when advancing your sleep with bright light. It's just that the psychological and social cues tending to delay your sleep become stronger as your sleep phase advances. You will have less and less time to finish dinner, attend to chores, respond to e-mail, and make phone calls before you must start getting ready for bed. You will need some time to develop new habits and routines, to erect a more impervious "buffer period" between your evening activities and bedtime, just like people who have never been night owls.

Once you are able to fall asleep at your targeted bedtime, you may not need any special morning light exposure to maintain your early weekday pattern. It is still a good idea to get such exposure on weekend mornings, after you have allowed yourself your one hour of extra sleep, to counter the incipient phase shift in your circadian rhythms that this oversleeping triggers. However, if you are among the many people with a delayed sleep phase who must constantly re-

sist a strong drift toward later bedtimes, you would benefit from receiving morning light even on weekdays, perhaps in a shorter stint
of fifteen to twenty minutes. It is crucial that you do not allow yourself to oversleep by more than one hour, even if you had gone to bed
very late that night. Your circadian system is hankering to drift later
at its first opportunity, and it will sweep you back "downstream" if
given the chance.

A major issue arising when bright light treatment is used to address severe difficulty falling asleep is that usually, the best time to
deliver light to advance the timing of sleep is in the morning hours,
when late sleepers would much rather be sleeping! As we write, we
are working with Professor Rea's group to develop a light mask that
could deliver light of sufficient intensity and of the proper blue
wavelengths through the closed eyelids of sleepers, hopefully without waking them up. If successful, this would allow light to be delivered shortly after the trough of the circadian temperature cycle,
when its effects would be most potent. There has been at least one
previous attempt to develop something similar; in this case, a mask
delivering white light through the eyelid produced a phase shift in
more severely delayed subjects but not in the experimental group as
a whole.

ANSWER: USE DARK OR BLUE-BLOCKING SUNGLASSES TO FILTER EVENING LIGHT

Recall that exposure to bright light in the evening or the first two-
thirds of the night tends to delay sleep rhythms. In the summer
months, when the sun sets much later and Daylight Savings Time
may be in effect, late evening light exposure tends to delay the sleep
patterns of everyone, whether they are particularly predisposed to

delayed sleep phase disorder or not. Teenagers are especially susceptible to a phase delay during this season, not only because their circadian clocks are more likely to "run slow," but also because they are
typically released from school obligations.

We may advise wearing wrap-around sunglasses to reduce light
exposure during summer evenings (in conjunction with morning
bright light treatment) when addressing severe cases of sleep phase
delay. With the discovery of the blue-sky sensitivity of the circadian
system described earlier, we are now recommending the use of
glasses that selectively block the blue portion of the light spectrum.
These glasses are available commercially—they have lenses that tint
the world an orange color. Although such glasses transmit more
light than standard sunglasses, we still caution against using them
when driving in the evening, as they may create unsafe visual conditions.

After you are safely home, you may need to wear your sunglasses
right up until you climb into bed and turn off your bedroom light. As
noted earlier, the lower levels of light exposure produced by artificial
lighting can still have circadian phase-shifting effects. This potential
source or disruption exists, of course, year round. Wearing orange-
tinted wrap-around glasses may make everything in your home look
a bit ghastly (and yourself a bit silly), but they can permit reading or
staring into a computer screen without eyestrain so long as sufficient
light intensity of longer wavelengths (the red-orange-yellow portion
of the spectrum) is getting through.

Recently, we have begun to use blue-blocking glasses in a way
that might seem counterintuitive to those of you who have been following our discussion of circadian rhythm phase shifts closely. Sometimes, we have teenagers who must meet a very early school bus
wear the glasses *in the morning*, while walking to the bus stop, wait-

ing for the bus, and—if teasing is not a problem—right up to the door of their school.

Why would we want to filter out blue light in the morning? We realized that some teenagers may have sleep phases that are so delayed, when they are pulled from bed and rushed out to the bus stop (especially at the start or end of the traditional school year, when it is still quite light before 7 or 7:30 A.M.), they may be receiving bright light exposure *before* the trough of their circadian temperature cycles. These students' harried parents may be exacerbating the problem—making it more likely that their children will sleep *later* on subsequent nights—in striving to get them to school on time.

How can we tell when the circadian temperature trough is occurring? To do this precisely, as required by research protocols, involves protracted laboratory procedures. Clinically, we can get a rough idea with simpler methods. As a rule of thumb, the temperature trough occurs slightly more than two hours before one's typical spontaneous wake-up time. For example, if your teenage son can *consistently* sleep to 11 A.M. when given the chance (not just for one or two days of recovery sleep), his temperature trough is likely occurring somewhat before 9 A.M. It's a good bet, therefore, that when he goes outside to wait for a bus around 7 A.M., this bright-light exposure is coming before his circadian temperature trough and will have a phase-delaying effect.

After discussions of delayed sleep phase syndrome and its treatment with Chronotherapy or bright light therapy, the question we are most often asked is, "Will I have to spend the rest of my life on such a rigid schedule for this to work?" The short answer is no. You will be able to have late nights now and then without falling back to square one. If "late" for you used to mean to 6 A.M., you may need to revise your thinking and head home at 2 A.M. Oversleeping may mean arising at 9 A.M. rather than in the mid-afternoon, and only on one weekend morning rather than both of them. Most important, you need to get right back on schedule after indulging in some extra sleep, supplemented by bright-light treatment. If you take advantage of a week's vacation to return to your old nocturnal ways, you will indeed need to reset your circadian clock. Even in this worse-case scenario, however, you will at least have the knowledge that such a shift has been accomplished before, and it will not seem nearly so daunting if required once again.

●   ●   ●

The Insomnia Answers presented in this chapter, addressing the various ways in which you might have difficulty falling asleep, should bring you all to the very threshold of that state. Regardless of the twists and turns of your particular treatment path, once at this threshold, you will all face the same challenge: *to complete the journey, your mind must not lodge an objection.* Turn now to Chapter 9. There, you will learn how to ease your mind's concerns and free yourself to sleep.

DIFFERENTIATE YOUR THERAPY—DIFFICULTY FALLING ASLEEP

Problem: Sunday Night Insomnia
Answer: Limit weekend oversleeping.

Problem: It usually takes an hour to fall asleep.
Answer: Maintain a "buffer period" between stimulating activities and bedtime.
Answer: Set aside "worry time" to address problems before you get into bed.
Answer: Follow Stimulus Control Instructions: retrain rapid sleep onset by using the bed only for sleep or sex and getting out of bed if you have been unable to fall asleep for twenty minutes.
Answer: Use melatonin three to four hours before the time you typically fall asleep.
Answer: Use Guided Imagery to shepherd your thoughts toward a peaceful place.
Answer: Exercise four to six hours before bedtime.
Answer: Take a hot bath about three hours before bedtime.

Problem: It usually takes several hours to fall asleep.
Answer: Maintain a consistent weekday rising time; limit weekend oversleeping to one hour.
Answer: Chronotherapy: rotate your bedtime progressively later around the clock.
Answer: Bright light treatment: obtain at least thirty minutes of bright light exposure *after you awaken*. (See text for timing details.)
Answer: Use dark or blue-blocking sunglasses to filter *evening* light.
Answer: Use melatonin three to four hours before the time you typically fall asleep.

CHAPTER SEVEN

Answers for Difficulty Staying Asleep

Suddenly finding yourself awake in the middle of the night brings a special exasperation beyond what might be expected from other forms of insomnia. To your mind, you did everything right. You put in a full day. It was all you could do to fend off sleep after dinner—you could have easily extended the short snooze you allowed yourself then. Instead, you waited until bedtime, settled yourself down once more, and fell asleep without a hitch. At that point, sleep was out of your hands. You should have been able to glide to a gentle landing in the morning without further effort, like a kid on a slide. Instead, sleep left you awkwardly stranded partway through.

Glancing at your alarm clock, you can hardly believe it is only three in the morning. Bleary-eyed, you might transfer to the couch, so as not to disturb your bed partner with tossing and turning. You may repair to a recliner to watch reruns or plow through a thriller. You could get an early start on answering your e-mail. Or you might just stay in bed, trying to remain as still as possible and, if you're lucky, pick up an hour or so of additional sleep. No matter how you choose to fill the expanse of wakefulness that looms ahead, there is little doubt that you are contending with our second category of insomnia, difficulty staying asleep. If there is a silver lining to this grim picture, it is that numerous treatments are available that can help fill more of your night with sleep.

Problem: You Awaken After a Few Hours of Sleep

Suppose your Sleep Log looks like the one that follows, confirming that for you, getting to sleep is not a problem, but staying asleep is. You can generally count on falling asleep within fifteen or twenty minutes but consistently awaken for no apparent reason three or four hours later. Subsequent sleep is short-lived, if it occurs at all. You are left with just time on your hands for the remainder of the night, occasionally getting in a little more sleep just before your alarm goes off.

Morning's Date	Time to Fall Asleep	Amount of Sleep	Fatigue Rating 1 Lo–10 Hi
Mo 3/16	15 min.	4 hrs	3
Tu 3/17	15 min.	4 1/2 hrs	5
We 3/18	20 min.	4 1/2 hrs	7
Th 3/19	10 min.	5 1/4 hrs	6
Fr 3/20	5 min.	5 1/2 hrs	8
Sat 3/21	5 min.	6 1/2 hrs	7
Sun 3/22	30 min.	5 1/2 hrs	5

ANSWER: STIMULUS CONTROL INSTRUCTIONS

Whether you abandon your bed in favor of various nocturnal diversions or remain ensnared in a twist of blankets and sheets, eventually your mind and body will come to expect wakefulness rather than sleep at night. You will have made a habit of not sleeping in bed. An effective way to break this habit is to re-train your expectations with Stimulus Control Instructions. We discussed the rationale for this well-validated treatment in the previous chapter when addressing difficulty falling asleep. Because Stimulus Control Instructions strengthen the association between being in bed and actually falling asleep, the treatment is also quite useful for those of you who have become conditioned to expect a prolonged awakening in the middle of the night. We will, therefore, repeat here the Stimulus Control Instructions as we apply them:

1. If you are not asleep within about twenty minutes, *get out of bed.*

2. Don't get back into bed until you are sleepy or feel you can fall asleep.

3. Once in bed, repeat step 1.

4. Do not use the bed for anything besides sleep and sex.

5. Wake up at the same time every weekday. (You can sleep an hour later on weekends.)

6. Don't nap.

When you get out of bed, you should occupy yourself with light reading rather than engaging in anything too challenging or engrossing. As during the "buffer period," avoid becoming too physically or mentally active. Instead, sit quietly, waiting for a wave of sleepiness to wash over you. Don't worry about missing an opportunity to get back to sleep right away—you've probably experienced plenty of worse nights. In fact, you're not likely to lose much sleep at all but will merely substitute peaceful reading or listening in a chair for tossing and turning in bed.

ANSWER: SEEK EVALUATION AND TREATMENT FOR DEPRESSION

As we learned in Chapter 3, persistent early morning awakenings are a hallmark of depression. This mood disturbance is characterized by an overall shift in the distribution of REM sleep into earlier hours of the night, beginning with its initial appearance, which may come perhaps forty or fifty minutes after sleep onset, as opposed to a more typical latency of about an hour and a half. REM sleep normally makes up a large percentage of sleep in the early morning. In depressed individuals who have phase-advanced REM sleep, these last hours of the night are more likely to be filled with wakefulness.

If you tend to awaken too early in the morning and your Zung Self-Rating Depression Scale documented such symptoms as hopelessness, tearfulness, irritability, or loss of appetite, it is reasonable to assume that your sleep disturbance is at least in part secondary to mood disorder. Directly addressing your depression—whether by pharmacotherapy, psychotherapy, or both in combination—should enable you to enjoy more prolonged sleep periods. This strategy is more likely to lead to stable sleep improvement than would the use of sleeping pills to extend sleep while leaving underlying affective disturbance untreated.

ANSWER: SET ASIDE "WORRY TIME" AND MAINTAIN A "BUFFER PERIOD"

Early morning awakenings can be the result of getting into bed with an unresolved conflict, or simply with too much pent-up excitement.

This may seem counterintuitive—if you were able to fall asleep without too much problem, wouldn't that imply that you successfully wound down for the night? Not necessarily. As we learned in Chapter 2, the Sleep Drive is quite high at bedtime, having built up across an entire day of wakefulness. The pull that this drive exerts in the first hours of the night can override, at least temporarily, considerable agitation.

The first hours of sleep typically contain our entire allotment of Slow Wave Sleep, the deepest NREM stages notable for their high arousal threshold. We are very difficult to fully awaken while in Slow Wave Sleep, regardless of whether we are harboring internal commotion or exposed to environmental disturbances. When our Slow Wave Sleep has run its course, we alternate between lighter NREM sleep and progressively longer REM periods. These stages may be punctuated with brief arousals. Now those unresolved worries we have taken to bed have their chance to wreak havoc. Every transient arousal gives the mind a few seconds' opportunity to latch onto some distressing thought, which can then be used as a wedge to pry apart sleep.

The foregoing explains why some of the same interventions that we introduced for people suffering from difficulty falling asleep can also be helpful for those whose primary problem is staying asleep. Setting aside "worry time" to identify and at least temporarily resolve potentially intrusive issues prevents them from resurfacing in the middle of the night, when they are more likely to break apart your sleep. Similarly, maintaining a "buffer period" in which to disengage from the day's events blocks them from disrupting your slumber. Both interventions restrict the flow of worrisome thoughts that would otherwise serve to fuel your racing mind. Consult the sections on worry time and the buffer period in Chapter 6 for a more detailed discussion of these treatments.

ANSWER: USE BRIGHT LIGHT TO DELAY YOUR SLEEP PHASE

Early morning awakenings can also result from a circadian rhythm disturbance known as advanced sleep phase disorder, which is the mirror of the delayed sleep phase type. In this disorder, the temperature and hormonal rhythms that underlay our sleep propensity are shifted earlier, to such an extent that sleep often arrives inadvertently after dinner, typically while watching television from a couch or easy chair. If sleep has its onset by 8 or 9 P.M., it is not surprising that by 3 or 4 A.M. it has run its course. While a delayed sleep phase is typically seen in adolescents and young adults, advanced sleep phase disorder is more often seen in the elderly.

Early morning awakenings reflecting an underlying phase advance are effectively treated with bright-light exposure, this time applied in the evening hours. As the light is being received *before* the trough of the temperature cycle, its effect will be to delay the sleep rhythm. A greater duration of exposure is generally required, because the light is being received six or so hours before the temperature cycle has reached its nadir, when its phase shifting effect is weaker. Fortunately, it is relatively easy to sit by a bright light device for an hour or longer in the evening while watching television or reading, compared to the difficulty of getting in even thirty minutes of exposure during the morning rush.

Let's consider a scenario in which you have been falling asleep inadvertently before 9 P.M. and waking around 3 A.M. You are aiming to shift your bedtime to 10 P.M. You might start by obtaining an hour of bright-light exposure from 8:30 to 9:30 P.M., which would leave you thirty minutes to get yourself ready for bed. During this hour, you could engage in quiet activities appropriate to a buffer period. Although bright light often has an alerting effect, you should still take care not to doze off while seated. It would be better to interrupt your light exposure by getting up and moving around if necessary to avoid falling asleep even for just a few minutes. If you begin to notice that, contrary to your previous history, you are beginning to experience some difficulty *falling* asleep, you may want to start your light exposure thirty or sixty minutes earlier or limit its duration to half an hour.

Your goal is to give yourself just enough push with bright light to make it through your evening drowsiness. When you arrive at your targeted bedtime, you can then allow yourself to glide down into sleep. With repeated exposure, your sleep phase will begin to shift later, so you will eventually find it easier to stay awake in the evening, even when you are not able to undergo light treatment.

A key notion to understand is that bright light treatment in the evening can help you sleep more consistently through the night— regardless of whether your morning awakenings stem directly from a circadian phase advance or from one of the other causes we have been considering, such as cognitive hyperarousal or major depression. Therefore, you do not have to be certain as to the exact cause of your sleep disturbance to benefit from this therapy. If you can identify a persistent pattern from your Sleep Logs indicating that your best sleep is likely to occur in the early part of the night, whereas you are likely to be awake well before morning, you can use evening light exposure to push your sleep later.

ANSWER: USE DARK OR BLUE-BLOCKING SUNGLASSES TO FILTER MORNING LIGHT

In the previous chapter, we discussed how bright light exposure obtained after the body temperature has reached its nadir tends to advance one's sleep phase. For people who have problems falling asleep at night and who tend to oversleep in the morning, this effect of morning light is therapeutic. In your case, however, such light exposure will make matters worse—you are already awakening too early! Therefore, you would benefit from wearing dark or blue-blocking sunglasses for the first several hours after you first awaken. This is especially important if you go outside, but it may also be helpful when you stay indoors with the lights on (or sit in front of a bright computer screen) following your early awakening. Blue-blocking lenses are preferable for such indoor activities, as they allow more light to reach the eye without triggering a shift in the timing of sleep.

ANSWER: USE HYPNOTIC MEDICATION TO PROLONG SLEEP

We believe that nondrug treatments are generally preferable for the treatment of insomnia. They are as effective as medications (as confirmed by well-controlled research studies) and avoid a host of problems that may be associated with drug use. We also believe that all else being equal, the quality of sleep obtained without drugs is superior to that of drug-induced sleep. That said, we acknowledge that some people with insomnia may require long-term use of hypnotic medication to sustain sleep.

We assume that the strength of the Sleep Drive varies across individuals, as does any trait, so that in most people it is moderately intense, in some particularly strong, and in others exceptionally weak. This latter group may require hypnotic medication to sleep through the night. Additionally, it appears that some people are more susceptible than others to weakening of their Sleep Drive with advancing age. In these cases, directly reinforcing sleep with medication over the long term may also be warranted.

How can you tell if you require a pharmacological boost to sleep well? It is difficult to assess the strength of your Sleep Drive directly, given the way it interacts with the Alerting Force and other factors to yield a given level of sleepiness. However, a number of clinical features, if present, would argue *against* taking sleeping pills.

Anxiety or Depression

To begin with, if you suspect that anxiety or depression are a part of your sleep disturbance, this should be addressed through cognitive behavioral treatment or appropriate medication *before* you and your physician consider long-term use of drugs specifically to strengthen your sleep. We have already discussed how treating depression should take priority when insomnia is present among its symptom cluster. In the case of anxiety disorder, some cognitive and behavioral therapies aimed at enhancing sleep may also address anxiety symptoms. However, if you and your physician feel that you need to take anti-anxiety medication, ask your doctor to consider a drug regimen that dampens anxiety throughout the day, and especially in the evening, as opposed to only at bedtime. By then, it is too late to wind down properly, and you are likely to experience a short night of sleep.

Excessive Daytime Sleepiness

If you are experiencing considerable daytime sleepiness together with restless sleep, you should discuss undergoing evaluation for physiologically based sleep disturbance with your doctor before opting for long-term medication. This scenario is consistent with significant sleep fragmentation, in which dozens or even hundreds of arousals, lasting just a few seconds each, repeatedly interrupt sleep continuity. Such fragmentation is often the result of sleep disordered breathing or repeated limb movements. Oftentimes, these transient arousals are not experienced as awakenings at all, but rather are collectively perceived as light, restless sleep.

Altered Timing of Sleep

If your Sleep Log demonstrates sleep of at least average duration, but a mismatch between when it occurs and when it should appear to best meet societal obligations, you would probably do better with a phase shift than with a pill.

Finally, if you sleep only four or five hours per night but are not especially sleepy during the daytime, you may just be a naturally short sleeper. Trying to extend your sleep pharmacologically in this case could well be counterproductive.

Choosing a Medication

If you have ruled out psychological distress, circadian rhythm disorder, physiologic disturbance, and environmental nuisance—yet your sleep seems to peter out after three or four hours—you may indeed benefit from some medication with sleep-maintaining properties. A wide range of agents are used for this purpose, including benzodiazepine and nonbenzodiazepine hypnotics, sedating antidepressants, and anticonvulsants. As discussed in Chapter 3, typical strategies for difficulty staying asleep include taking a sleeping pill at bedtime with a sufficient half-life to maintain sleep throughout the night, or alternatively, taking a very short-acting pill after awakening in the middle of the night to accumulate a few more hours of sleep. Nonprescription remedies including antihistamines, herbal preparations, and nutritional supplements are also employed, although with less consistent results.

All of these substances vary in their mechanism, duration of action, metabolism, compatibility with other medications and alcohol, side effect profile, and other important factors. Some have been subject to extensive testing under the purview of the federal Food and Drug Administration (FDA) to assess safety and efficacy. Some have undergone FDA scrutiny for other indications, and are used "off label" to treat insomnia, based on clinical experience. And some are wholly untested. For all of these reasons, the decision to use any hypnotic agent is one you should make in consultation with your physician.

• • •

The Insomnia Answers presented in this chapter, addressing the problem of difficulty staying asleep, should bring you all back to the very threshold of that state. Regardless of the twists and turns of your particular treatment path, once at this threshold, you will all face the same challenge: *to complete the journey, your mind must not lodge an objection.* Turn now to Chapter 9. There, you will learn how to ease your mind's concerns and free yourself to sleep.

DIFFERENTIATE YOUR THERAPY—DIFFICULTY STAYING ASLEEP

Problem: You have a prolonged awakening after just a few hours of sleep.

Answer: Follow Stimulus Control Instructions: retrain rapid sleep onset by using the bed only for sleep or sex and getting out of bed if you have been unable to fall asleep for twenty minutes.

Answer: Seek evaluation and treatment for depression if indicated by your Zung Self-Rating Depression Scale score.

Answer: Maintain a "buffer period" between stimulating activities and bedtime.

Answer: Set aside "worry time" to address problems before you get into bed.

Answer: Bright light treatment: obtain at least one hour of bright light exposure *before you go to bed*. (See text for timing details.)

Answer: Use dark or blue-blocking sunglasses to filter *morning* light.

Answer: Use hypnotic medication to prolong sleep.

Answer: Use Guided Imagery to shepherd your thoughts to a peaceful place.

Answer: Exercise four to six hours before bedtime.

Answer: Take a hot bath about three hours before bedtime.

CHAPTER EIGHT

Answers for Broken or Irregular Sleep

If you suffer from broken sleep, your problem is quite different from the other types of insomnia in a very important way: *you have no difficulty getting to sleep, whether at bedtime or in the middle of the night.* In fact, you may fall asleep three, five, or even ten times each night. This may seem like a hollow victory, but we do not make light of this achievement, and neither should you. It means you have the right mind-set to enter sleep. You are not inhibited from crossing the boundary between wakefulness and sleep and can do so repeatedly, even after your Sleep Drive has started to lose steam and your Alerting Force is beginning to rise. Your problem is that something is breaking the flow of your sleep each time you get it underway.

Another major contrast between you and those who have consistent difficulty falling asleep or staying asleep is that your sleep is likely to appear totally erratic. It may come in spurts of forty-five, sixty, or ninety minutes; on other occasions you might get a stretch of several hours. These segments taken together do not nearly cover the time you actually spend in bed, leaving cracks of arousal as well as gaping awakenings to repeatedly interrupt your sleep. You probably spend so much time and effort transitioning in and out of sleep that you are thoroughly exhausted by morning rather than refreshed. Broken sleep of this sort can be particularly demoralizing, as you never seem to manage an escape from the night's travails. If this pattern describes your experience, take heart; this chapter offers effective treatments formulated especially for you.

At first glance, it may be strange to be speaking here of sleep patterns at all, as if there could be distinct forms of chaos. Yet in fact there are subtle differences in the ways sleep can break apart. Appreciating these variations will help you differentiate your therapy and lead to more satisfying sleep.

Problem: Your Sleep Is Broken

The problem we will consider first is perhaps the most common. It is the case when time spent in bed is primarily confined to the nighttime hours, with occasional daytime napping. While the time allotted for bed is typically quite generous, perhaps extending well into the morning, sleep itself is meager.

Morning's Date	Time to Fall Asleep	Amount of Sleep	Fatigue Rating 1 Lo–10 Hi
Mo 8/2	90 min.	5 1/2 hrs	3
Tu 8/3	20 min.	6 hrs	8
We 8/4	60 min.	5 1/2 hrs	6
Th 8/5	120 min.	5 3/4 hrs	6
Fr 8/6	45 min.	7 1/2 hrs	7
Sat 8/7	5 min.	7 1/2 hrs	5
Sun 8/8	45 min.	6 3/4 hrs	4

If you have sleep of this sort, there indeed doesn't seem to be much of a pattern as to when episodes occur. Sometimes it takes you a long while to fall asleep; on other nights sleep will be established quickly, only to be interrupted by a prolonged awakening. Sometimes sleep seems cleaved evenly into hour-long segments, as if by a careful chef; at other times, it may resemble a mélange of chunks and tidbits. Occasionally, you will be surprised to slumber well into the morning, while at other times sleep will abandon you before the black night sky has even begun to fade.

How does such broken and erratic sleep come about? The answer has as much to do with the response to sleeplessness as with sleep itself: when poor sleepers find themselves contending with unreliable sleep on a chronic basis, they have a tendency to spend more time in bed, hoping to capture as much sleep as they can. This is one of the main Perpetuating practices maintaining insomnia, as we learned in Chapter 3. Sleep will then thin out, trying to cover the wider territory set aside for it, eventually tearing apart. The effect is analogous to the broadening of an oil spill on the ocean's surface. The oil starts out as a thick glob, but without containment, it spreads into an expansive slick and breaks up. Our bedraggled insomniacs may extend their bedtimes repeatedly, but in doing so, they do not generally accumulate more sleep. Instead, they only give their tattered sleep more room in which to disperse.

ANSWER: SLEEP RESTRICTION THERAPY

About twenty years ago, we introduced Sleep Restriction Therapy, a simple behavioral treatment for insomnia that works to reduce variability in the timing of sleep while increasing its depth. Dr. William Dement, one of the founders of Sleep Medicine, once called Sleep

Restriction Therapy the first "somnologic" treatment for insomnia, perhaps because it exploits sleep processes that had been discerned over the course of previous decades of sleep research. It had been learned, for example, that habitually "short sleepers"—those who only spend, say, five or six hours in bed—sleep efficiently, with very little bedtime given to wakefulness. Short sleepers also spend a greater percentage of their total sleep time in deepest Slow Wave Sleep and reduced percentages in light Stage 1 or moderately deep Stage 2 Non-REM sleep.

You already have some familiarity with Sleep Restriction Therapy, because a modified version formed part of the Preliminary Treatment we introduced in Chapter 5. If your sleep remains broken and haphazard, it is time to apply the treatment in its full strength.

Recall how we applied this modified treatment using the baseline Sleep Log you completed initially. Your average bedtime and rising time were estimated by splitting the cloud of circles delimiting the start and finish of each night in bed. In our current example, these bedtimes and rising times yield an average time in bed of nine hours. Next, the average amount of sleep you obtained was calculated by adding up the segments for each night, as well as daytime naps, summing across the week, and dividing by seven. In our exam-

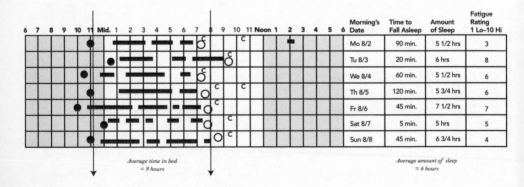

	Morning's Date	Time to Fall Asleep	Amount of Sleep	Fatigue Rating 1 Lo–10 Hi
	Mo 8/2	90 min.	5 1/2 hrs	3
	Tu 8/3	20 min.	6 hrs	8
	We 8/4	60 min.	5 1/2 hrs	6
	Th 8/5	120 min.	5 3/4 hrs	6
	Fr 8/6	45 min.	7 1/2 hrs	7
	Sat 8/7	5 min.	5 hrs	5
	Sun 8/8	45 min.	6 3/4 hrs	4

Average time in bed = 9 hours *Average amount of sleep = 6 hours*

ple, these sleep segments averaged across the week work out to six hours per night.

Our current version of Sleep Restriction Therapy is quite simple to implement. You may want to keep a new one-week Sleep Log to establish a current baseline. Once you have determined the average amount of sleep you think you obtain nightly, choose a consistent bedtime and rising time to yield *exactly* this amount of time in bed, so that *all* the excess wakefulness is wrung from your sleep schedule. (Recall that in our Preliminary Treatment, we directed you to restrict your bedtime so that only *half* of the wakefulness was cut from your schedule.) You may choose to shift your bedtime and rising time equally—albeit in opposite directions—to accomplish this, just as we did in our Preliminary Treatment. Or you may cut a bit more from one side than the other, giving yourself either extra time to wind down before going to bed or more time to prepare for the coming day. Avoid napping, even though daytime naps were originally counted when arriving at your average total sleep time. The resulting Sleep Log after applying SRT might, therefore, look like this:

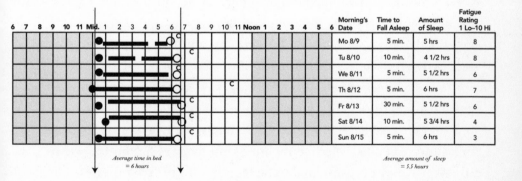

	Morning's Date	Time to Fall Asleep	Amount of Sleep	Fatigue Rating 1 Lo–10 Hi
	Mo 8/9	5 min.	5 hrs	8
	Tu 8/10	10 min.	4 1/2 hrs	8
	We 8/11	5 min.	5 1/2 hrs	6
	Th 8/12	5 min.	6 hrs	7
	Fr 8/13	30 min.	5 1/2 hrs	6
	Sat 8/14	10 min.	5 3/4 hrs	4
	Sun 8/15	5 min.	6 hrs	3

Average time in bed = 6 hours

Average amount of sleep = 5.5 hours

In this example, we have cut about an hour and a half from each side of the bedtime schedule. This way, our sleeper is not going to bed extremely late or getting out of bed way before the sun rises. The schedule yields six hours in bed, which matches the average amount of sleep obtained during the baseline week.

It is important to note that when instituting Sleep Restriction Therapy, we set a lower limit for the initial amount of time allotted in bed at five hours (one hour less than in our Preliminary Treatment). That is, even if the average amount of sleep you think you obtained on your baseline log was just three or four hours, you should still target five hours in bed. This way, you will at least garner a minimal amount of bed rest during the night along with any sleep you manage to accumulate.

Notice in our example that it takes a few nights before the six hours in bed have more or less filled with sleep. This is a common response. The first night or two on Sleep Restriction Therapy can indeed be rough, because you are aware that the night will be short, and this only adds to the anxiety about sleeping you are already bringing to bed. We ask you to bear with us for a short while. Remember, your sleep problems have probably been entrenched for years; they will take some time to respond to treatment. But if you can manage to pull yourself out of bed at the appointed hour, regardless of how much sleep you obtained during the night, and remain out of bed or off the couch all the next day, within a couple of nights, sleep will begin to extend through more of your allotted bedtime.

You are likely wondering how long you can be expected to stay on such a drastically shortened bedtime schedule. The answer is not forever, but it could be anywhere from one week to a month or more. You should keep to the schedule until your average amount of wakefulness per night is estimated to be less than forty-five minutes. The reasoning is this: even a good sleeper will often take about fifteen minutes to fall asleep, and one or two awakenings during the night of similar duration should be tolerable. On the other hand, if you're already spending forty-five minutes awake, you will probably not benefit from any more time in bed.

If you were sleeping five or more hours to begin with, you should have very little wakefulness remaining in your restricted bedtime schedule because we initially set it to exactly match your sleep time. After one week of intensive sleep consolidation, you will likely be able to start extending your bedtime, as described in the following paragraphs. If, however, you only logged three or four hours of sleep initially, it may take a while before you reach the threshold of forty-five minutes or less of wakefulness per night, given the relatively generous five hours you are still allowed in bed.

When you are sleeping most of your allotted bedtime, and your estimated wakefulness across the week averages under forty-five minutes per night, it's time to add fifteen minutes to your bedtime. If you are falling asleep within five or ten minutes of getting into bed, you can add the extra time to the beginning of the night by shifting your bedtime earlier. Otherwise, let yourself remain in bed fifteen minutes later in the morning. Once you make a choice, stick with it.

Repeat this adjustment as necessary, recording a full week of Sleep Log data at each new bedtime length before estimating the average amount of time you are spending awake nightly to see if you qualify for an additional fifteen minutes. "Fifteen minutes!" we can almost hear the groans, "what good will that do?" In fact, a couple of fifteen-minute extensions can go a long way toward improving the way you feel in the morning if you are able to reliably spend them asleep.

You are probably thinking that this claim hardly jibes with your experience. You can recall gaining or losing an hour of sleep without it making much difference at all in how you felt the next day, let alone fifteen or thirty minutes. You may feel you need to obtain that rarity, a full eight hours of sleep, before you perceive any benefit. One reason for this disparity is that your sleep pattern is so haphazard to begin with. When sleep is well regulated, the effects of relatively minor adjustments become more discernable. On the other hand, when the amount of sleep accumulated on any given night is highly variable, these effects tend to be lost.

A second reason for our optimism is that if you can get to the point of accumulating five hours of sleep on a consistent basis, you are already close to the amount of sleep most of us need to function passably the next day. We usually have considerable difficulty managing on five hours of sleep or less, while we can make do in a pinch with six hours, even if this amount is hardly optimal and over the long term will require extension. Somewhere in between five and six hours of sleep there is a tipping point. That is why, starting from a base of five hours of consolidated sleep, just a couple of fifteen-minute increments can be so effective.

In addition to the physiological regulation of sleep that Sleep Restriction Therapy promotes, it also brings a psychological benefit. The short night of sleep you will experience while undergoing treatment is different from the short nights you experienced beforehand. It is different because it is under your control. Insomnia brings disruption at many levels; however, one of its most pernicious effects is the feeling of helplessness it bestows. Do you remember from your grade school years how, when a playground wound required antiseptic or a stubborn Band-Aid needed replacement, it sometimes felt better to take matters into your own hands and apply the first aid yourself? It's not that the iodine didn't sting or that your skin didn't feel raw as you peeled off the dressing. It's just that when you took control, the experience was not quite so insufferable. The same is true with insomnia. You must still contend with extra waking hours, but because these hours have been intentionally slotted into an extended evening or to follow an earlier rising time, they no longer represent "sleeplessness" in quite the same way.

A major side effect of Sleep Restriction Therapy is daytime sleepiness. Use particular caution when driving or operating dangerous machinery during the first weeks of treatment. If you find that your sleep is consolidating quickly, or that the degree of daytime sleepiness you experience is difficult to tolerate, by all means modify your bedtime schedule by adding thirty minutes at a time during these first weeks; you can later "fine-tune" your sleep with fifteen-minute increments.

Problem: Your Sleep Is Scattered Around the Clock

Stella had lost track of time. She could still remember living a life measured out by the hour, with reliably alternating periods of activity and sleep. She used to see the sun on a regular basis and looked forward to fair weather so she could get in some rollerblading or tend to her garden. These memories were fading. Now, it seemed that there was little difference between day and night. Regardless of the hour, Stella was always too tired to work or play, yet too unsettled to sleep.

She had consulted a slew of specialists, practitioners of alternative medicine as well as mainstream physicians. Her doctors had checked for thyroid dysfunction, nutritional deficiencies, Lyme Disease, AIDS and other infections, as well as for various neurological disorders. Some settled on Chronic Fatigue Syndrome; others were not convinced she met formal diagnostic criteria for that condition. Stella had undergone batteries of tests and had been tried on a long list of antidepressant medications, anxiolytics, stimulant drugs, and nutritional supplements—all with equivocal results. She had all but given up on finding a name for her ailment and wasn't even sure it mattered anymore. She just wanted to feel better, to keep the rest of her once-active life from slipping from her grasp.

Before appearing for consultation, Stella had been asked to fill out a Sleep Log. She protested at first that she had no pattern to depict—and that furthermore, she could barely differentiate between hours spent awake and asleep. Nonetheless, Stella was asked to make her best guess—she was told that just demonstrating the lack of a pattern could potentially be useful. And in fact, the haphazard scattering of naps Stella rendered across the log not only testified to her dilemma, it was also the starting point for restructuring her life.

6 7 8 9 10 11 Mid. 1 2 3 4 5 6 7 8 9 10 11 Noon 1 2 3 4 5 6	Morning's Date	Time to Fall Asleep	Amount of Sleep	Fatigue Rating 1 Lo–10 Hi
	Mo 10/10	45 min.	8 1/2 hrs	5
	Tu 10/11	30 min.	7 1/2 hrs	5
	We 10/12	90 min.	7 1/4 hrs	6
	Th 10/13	90 min.	5 1/2 hrs	7
	Fr 10/14	30 min.	8 1/2 hrs	6
	Sat 10/15	15 min.	9 hrs	6
	Sun 10/16	30 min.	6 hrs	6

ANSWER: RESERVE TIME FOR WAKEFULNESS INSTEAD OF SLEEP

People contending with chronic illness often end up with haphazard sleep such as Stella's. They are caught in a bind, where they may require significant amounts of bed rest to promote healing or to counter pain and fatigue. Yet this extra time spent either sleeping, trying to sleep, or just resting encourages sleep to fragment and scatter around the clock. A similar problem occurs in those who are wheelchair bound. With limited physical activity and nearly every hour spent sitting, reclining, or in bed, the sleep-wake cycle tends to break down to the point where alertness is absent much of the day, while deep sleep is nowhere to be found at night.

If you have an irregular sleep pattern developed in the context of chronic illness or disability, it would be presumptuous for us to recommend that you keep regular bedtimes, yielding eight hours in bed at night, while staying completely out of bed as well as off the couch by day. Such mainstream advice has likely been proffered on numerous occasions. When you tried to follow it, the results were predictable: your sleep remained broken and limited at night, leading to overwhelming fatigue as you attempted to avoid resting during the daytime, even to the point of exacerbating your condition.

Rather than trying to directly corral sleep as with Sleep Restriction Therapy, a better strategy would be to generate a new sleep-wake rhythm by building upon gradually expanding "wakeful zones." We assume that initially, you will require considerable time resting or napping during the day, in part due to your physical condition, and also because your sleep is so poorly consolidated at night. Our goal will be to gradually reduce this amount. We need to strike the right balance between the amount of rest needed to feel your best during waking hours and the amount of activity required to best consolidate nocturnal sleep.

We start by asking that you choose just two hours in the morning and two hours in the evening when you will do your utmost to avoid sleeping or even resting. It is very important that these hours remain constant from day to day. They should include as much physical activity and, in the case of the morning zone, daylight exposure as possible. Try to schedule appointments and other obligations during your designated morning zone to better help you adhere to your schedule. For a similar reason, the evening zone is a good time to make social engagements. You may find that getting out of the house for short forays can be invigorating, as opposed to more fatiguing extended excursions. In any case, to the extent that you can spend some time away from home, there will be that much less potential for excessive time in bed to accumulate.

You are not required to spend all the hours in between your two wakeful zones in bed. By all means, try to remain as active as possible throughout the day. We are simply suggesting that when you *do* find it necessary to rest, you should plan these rest periods to take place outside a wakeful zone.

After a few weeks, add a half-hour increment to one zone, and a few weeks later add an extra half hour to the other. Continue in this fashion until you've opened up three to four hours for waking activity in each zone, as much as you can comfortably handle. At this point, you may want to open up yet a third wakeful zone, this time in the afternoon. Start with a short, two-hour window and gradually add to it as before, taking care to maintain adequate rest in between your hopefully burgeoning zones of activity.

With the log's representation of her chaotic existence as a starting point, we began by asking Stella to carve out hours when she agreed to refrain from even trying to sleep. She hesitated to designate two wakeful zones at first, but she did agree to a single three-hour zone in the morning from 9 A.M. to noon. We recommended Stella go outdoors for exposure to daylight as much as she could during these hours. During the other twenty-one hours of the day and night, she was free to catch up on sleep or rest on an as-needed basis.

Stella began to have confidence that her morning energy level could be counted on to run short errands or schedule visits to doctors. After a few weeks, we inserted another two-hour wakeful zone in her schedule, this time in the early evening. Stella discovered that it was indeed easier to leave the house then, so she wouldn't be tempted to lie down. In the months that followed, her two designated active zones were gradually expanded to three and a half hours apiece. What was even more heartening, Stella was beginning to sleep more soundly at night. She never worked up to much beyond six hours of sleep punctuated by a few short interruptions, and she continued to require two scheduled daytime rest periods lasting about ninety minutes apiece. Nonetheless, Stella had built up a sleep/wake cycle she could live with.

As the admittedly extreme example provided by Stella suggests, we can work with lots of variations on the theme of sleep, including patterns containing regular naps if required. However, most of our readers who are not contending with debilitating conditions would do well to avoid napping, at least during the treatment phase, as they strive to reposition and consolidate their sleep. Furthermore, all but a few of those who feel they must nap from the outset should be able to get by with a single nap per twenty-four-hour cycle. The nap should be less than an hour, planned as opposed to inadvertent, and completed at least nine hours before bedtime. An important exception to this rule is made for night and rotating shift workers, who may require a more prolonged nap prior to their work shift and consequently a less pronounced discrepancy between the duration of their main sleep period and that of their supplementary nap.

Problem: You Awaken About Every Ninety Minutes

Are the awakenings depicted on your Sleep Logs spaced evenly about an hour and a half apart? You may think you are the only hapless sleeper whose awakenings can be relied upon to set a clock, but in fact, you have lots of company.

	Morning's Date	Time to Fall Asleep	Amount of Sleep	Fatigue Rating 1 Lo–10 Hi
	Mo 4/26	5 min.	6 hrs	4
	Tu 4/27	5 min.	6 hrs	6
	We 4/28	30 min.	6 1/2 hrs	6
	Th 4/29	20 min.	5 1/2 hrs	7
	Fr 4/30	0 min.	7 hrs	4
	Sat 5/1	5 min.	7 hrs + 1/4 hr	4
	Sun 5/2	0 min.	7 hrs	2

What's going on here? Typically, this pattern results when something is interfering with REM sleep, which normally appears about every ninety minutes across the night as part of the NREM/REM cycle. Oftentimes, some type of sleep-disordered breathing such as Obstructive Sleep Apnea is the culprit, because this disorder may be exacerbated in REM to the point where it is hard to maintain sleep at all in that stage. Most people who are diagnosed with Obstructive Sleep Apnea first come to clinical attention complaining of excessive daytime sleepiness, but for some, the disorder can present as a problem of sleep maintenance insomnia.

ANSWER: SCREEN FOR REM SLEEP DISORDERED BREATHING

If this pattern seems familiar to you, you may want to ask your bed partner (or, if you generally sleep alone, the next person who has occasion to observe you sleep) whether you tend to snore loudly, appear to pause in your breathing, or seem to be struggling for breath. If your problem is indeed confined primarily to REM sleep, your observer may have to wait an hour and a half or so to first observe it. Alternatively, you might arrange to have your sleep observed in the early morning hours, when REM sleep is more prominent. If such symptoms are confirmed, you should speak with your physician. Ultimately, consultation with a sleep specialist and overnight polysomnography may be required to establish the diagnosis.

ANSWER: REVIEW YOUR USE OF ALCOHOL AND MEDICATIONS

While alcohol can hasten sleep onset and indeed increase the amount of Slow Wave Sleep you accumulate during the first few hours of the night, it is a potent REM sleep suppressant and can give rise to the intermittent awakening pattern we have been considering during subsequent hours. Antidepressants and opioids are also known to suppress REM sleep. With regard to antidepressants, virtually complete suppression may be maintained for months or years on monoamine oxidase inhibitors, and chronic partial suppression is often seen on tricyclics as well as newer serotonin-specific reuptake inhibitors. Typically, patients using such antidepressants may have altered sleep architecture but not experience overt awakenings. However, there are exceptions, so if you are continuing to have sleep maintenance difficulties while on an antidepressant, you should consult with your doctor. Side effects of drugs can be so idiosyncratic that sometimes switching to another medication—even within the same class of drug—can bring about marked improvement.

ANSWER: CALM YOUR DREAMS

Larry psyched himself up for sleep as if it were a grueling prize fight. Each night, the match pitting Larry against his own dreams would last round after round, leaving him exhausted. They were all about being pursued, struggling with assailants, groping in the dark for a knife before an intruder found it first. Oftentimes, the same dream would recur, with minor variations, night after night. Even those that were relatively benign carried a tinge of frustration, as when he roamed the rows of a parking lot searching unsuccessfully for his car.

Sometimes the dream violence would propel Larry right out of his sleep. His body would feel as if it had just thawed, his mind jarred and confused. He could hardly move his limbs, but inside his heart was pounding. Other times, Larry's struggles stayed submerged under the lightest wash of sleep. He was somehow aware that he was dreaming, but still powerless to stop or even deflect the action. He had to take every hit before his alarm finally signaled an end to the night.

Given that sleepers experience REM sleep as vivid, movielike dreaming, it is not surprising that it is susceptible to interruption when dream content is particularly distressing. How dreams draw their themes and assume their forms has of course been the subject of intense speculation from many quarters—a discussion that is beyond the scope of our work. Anxiety dreams appear across a wide range of psychological circumstances. They can arise in sleepers who do not feel particularly anxious by day or agitated at bedtime. At the other extreme, they are a hallmark of patients contending with Post-Traumatic Stress Disorder.

Regardless of context, treatments are available that can help soothe anxiety dreams. Foremost among these is Imagery Rehearsal Therapy, developed by Krakow and colleagues. In this treatment, nightmare sufferers first collect their disturbing dreams in a journal. They then revise the dreams by splicing on new, more favorable or "masterful" endings. Each reworked scenario thus retains elements of the original nightmare as well as a more comforting outcome. These scenarios are repeatedly rehearsed during waking hours, for fifteen minutes or so at a time. Imagery Rehearsal Therapy has been shown to decrease the frequency of nightmares as well as improve sleep quality in general. Traditional cognitive behavioral treatments such as Relaxation Training and Systematic Desensitization have also demonstrated usefulness in this regard.

Problem: You Work a Variable Shift— No Set Work or Sleep Schedule

"It's like a giant video game," Cynthia explained. "Every time a maintenance guy has to walk the track, I enter his position into the computer and hold the local trains so he doesn't get run down. And then there are the crossings—you have to make sure that a train doesn't meet a truck at grade. When the express comes through, I've got to check who I have out there and get them out of the way. It's a lot to keep in mind, especially when I'm working on just a few hours of sleep. Look at this crazy schedule: two days off, then three afternoon shifts, a day off, then two days on, two days off, one night on, and then a double shift starting at 3 P.M. when I cover for my buddy."

Cynthia explained that despite her fourteen years on the railroad, she still didn't have nearly the seniority needed to work straight days. She probably could work a straight second shift, and she certainly could have the night shift, but then she would hardly ever see her husband, who had to leave for work by 7:30 in the morning. The railroad did not rotate workers through shifts in a scheduled progression. Cynthia's solution was to bid on jobs that filled in for absent workers and use up her vacation time to avoid nights as best she could.

Staying alert once she was on the job and the adrenalin started flowing did not present much of an issue. Her problem was falling asleep and staying asleep once back home. It seemed that Cynthia's sleep had dried up, leaving only puddles of naps strewn haphazardly across day and night. Following a day shift, Cynthia took an extended nap after dinner and then was up much of the night, finally falling asleep an hour or two before her alarm rang. When she worked second shift, Cynthia arrived home too wired to wind down for hours. After working nights, conking out at 8 A.M. from sheer exhaustion was

Morning's Date	Time to Fall Asleep	Amount of Sleep	Fatigue Rating 1 Lo–10 Hi
Mo 2/6	5 min.	6 hrs	5
Tu 2/7	5 min.	6 + 1 hrs	5
We 2/8	120 min.	5 hrs	7
Th 2/9	120 min.	5 1/2 hrs	6
Fr 2/10	90 min.	5 1/2 hrs	6
Sat 2/11	30 min.	6 1/2 hrs	5
Sun 2/12	75 min.	5 1/2 hrs + 2 hrs	5

Morning's Date	Time to Fall Asleep	Amount of Sleep	Fatigue Rating 1 Lo–10 Hi
Mo 2/13	60 min.	6 hrs + 1 1/2 hrs	5
Tu 2/14	75 min.	6 hrs	5
We 2/15	1 min.	4 hrs + 2 1/2 hrs	7
Th 2/16	1 min.	5 1/4 hrs	9

easy enough, but Cynthia could never sleep until noon, even if she managed to avoid being awakened by the phone or doorbell.

To the extent that Cynthia was compelled to work all three shifts, she was in fact asking too much of her sleep. Jumping from one shift to another flattened her circadian rhythms, leaving her partially alert most of the time, suspended in a borderline state that had to be roused fully awake by excitement or caffeine, or coaxed into sleep through inactivity, alcohol, or pills. Fortunately, Cynthia's goal of avoiding the night shift did allow us to bring some semblance of order to her schedule and more sleep into her allotted bedtimes.

ANSWER: ANCHOR SLEEP

We started by introducing "anchor sleep" into Cynthia's schedule. Anchor sleep is a concept derived from research protocols exploring the effects of various sleep schedules on circadian rhythms. It was found that when sleep was obtained at random times, underlying temperature and hormonal rhythms uncoupled from the twenty-four-hour clock and began to "free-run"—that is, they cycled with period lengths longer than twenty-four hours, as dictated by the internal circadian pacemaker. However, when sleep was consistently accumulated during a specific four-hour block (whether during the day or the night) and supplemented with sporadic naps, the underlying temperature and hormonal rhythms become re-entrained or "anchored" to the twenty-four-hour clock.

Anchor sleep of course could not be instituted if Cynthia worked around the clock—there would never be a four-hour block consistently available for sleep. However, when she primarily worked just the first and second shifts, she could maintain a late bedtime of about 12:30 A.M. on each of her work days as well as on her days off. This meant she could potentially sleep during the same five to six hours every night. We had seen from inspection of Cynthia's Sleep Logs that she was hardly ever successful at sleeping before 12:30 A.M., even when she had the chance, given the sleep phase-delaying effect of working the second and third shifts. We suggested that she take a brief nap soon after returning home from the day shift to hold off her main sleep period until 12:30 A.M. We also had Cynthia avoid sleeping late on days where she worked the second shift, moving her rising time (which had varied between 8:30 A.M. to 10:30 A.M.) to about 7:30 A.M. so she would be more likely to fall asleep at 12:30 A.M. the following night. She followed the same 12:30 A.M. to 7:30 A.M. schedule on her days off, supplemented as needed with a brief mid-day nap.

One caveat was required: as Cynthia's sleep/wake pattern began to stabilize around her block of anchor sleep, she felt more out of synch than ever when she had to work an occasional night shift. Late night was now devoted consistently to sleep when Cynthia was at home, and so her newly tuned circadian physiology pushed her toward more overt sleepiness when on the job during these hours. Cynthia was still able to fortify herself with coffee and get through the shift, just as most of us have experienced when occasionally compelled to stay awake at night. In fact, Cynthia reported that she seemed to have "more reserves" in this regard than formerly. This might have been because while Cynthia's clock-based Alerting Force was working more strongly against her at night, her homeostatic Sleep Drive was not augmented by as much sleep loss on her new schedule.

Problem: You Work a Night Shift

Apart from variable and rotating shifts, the other type of shift work that typically leads to insomnia (as well as a host of other complaints including fatigue, headaches, and gastrointestinal distress) is straight night shift work. This is due in part to the nearly universal tendency of night shift workers to rejoin the schedules of family and friends when not working—shopping, exercising, and socializing by day while sleeping as much as they can during their few nights off. Because of this repeated cycling between workday and weekend sleep patterns, the sleep of straight night shift workers begins to resemble that of variable or rotating shift workers, even if their work hours remain steady. The problems encountered by night shift workers also appear to stem from the relative lack of light exposure they get overall, as they sleep during some of the brightest hours of the day. Finally, there is the special challenge of sleeping against the cacophony of an awakening outside world, complete with serenading birds, honking commuters, chipper news anchors, and jingling cell phones.

ANSWER: WEAR DARK OR BLUE-BLOCKING SUNGLASSES IN THE MORNING

Strategies to help night shift workers better adapt to their working conditions have been the focus of attention from the sleep research community. The problem here is the reverse of what we encountered with delayed sleep phase disorder: in the case of night shift workers, we want to *foster* a phase delay so alertness is maximized during nocturnal work hours and consolidated sleep is extended through the morning and into the afternoon. The main culprit preventing this phase delay from occurring is morning sunlight. Night shift workers are typically exposed to bright light on their commute home, and bright light will also infiltrate the bedrooms of the ill prepared. If you are a night shift worker, your first defense against broken, restless sleep is, therefore, a pair of dark (or blue-blocking) sunglasses. Put these on before you step outside your workplace, and do not take them off until you get into bed.

Why is this so important, you might ask? After all, you've just worked a full shift; it would seem you should be able to sleep without too much difficulty. The problem is that although your body temperature minimum did begin to drift later with your return to work following a few nights off, it is still positioned too early to allow anything but fitful sleep in the daytime. Your temperature trough is likely suspended somewhere between the 4 to 5 A.M. position that characterizes typical nocturnal sleep (the pattern you probably followed last weekend) and the noon to 1 P.M. position that would allow you to sleep through a good part of today. Therefore, although you can manage to get to sleep in the morning due to the buildup of your Sleep Drive, your Alerting Force is working to wake you up right from the start.

Wearing dark or blue-blocking glasses from the workplace to your home (only after sunrise, of course—not if it is still dark outside!) will enable your temperature minimum to shift progressively later into the day as you work through the week. This in turn will allow you to sleep later into the day if you are not otherwise interrupted. You should help maintain this circadian shift by keeping very late bedtime hours during your time off, even if you allow some sleep to occur at night. Consider a 2 A.M. or 3 A.M. bedtime, with a rising time in mid-morning.

ANSWER: NAP BEFORE YOUR SHIFT

Many night shift workers eventually come to the discovery that nothing forestalls sleepiness on the job better than napping beforehand. That simple insight has now received ample backing from the research laboratory. While it may be somewhat more difficult to counter the effects of an Alerting Force that stubbornly clings to a diurnal pattern, dealing with a Sleep Drive that has been gathering steam across the day is more straightforward: sleeping, even for just an hour or two, will dissipate the Sleep Drive to a significant degree, so sleepiness will be less bothersome during enforced nocturnal wakefulness. Given that many night shift workers have a hard time sleeping seven or eight hours when they first come home from work, evening napping brings the additional benefit of limiting the accrual of sleep debt.

ANSWER: OBTAIN BRIGHT LIGHT EXPOSURE AT WORK

Bright light is the enemy of sleep in the morning, but it can help maintain alertness and entrain a delayed sleep phase when obtained during the night. Researchers have confirmed that bright light of about 3,000 lux delivered intermittently during the first six hours of a night shift tends to delay the core body temperature minimum into the morning hours, when night shift workers are attempting to sleep. In workplaces where little movement is required, this light exposure can be gained through use of a standard light box. In other settings, the support of facilities management must be enlisted to adjust lighting across a wide area. A cadre of consultants has sprung up to convince operations executives of the wisdom of such an investment, in terms of employee health, safety, and productivity.

ANSWER: PROTECT YOUR SLEEP FROM DAYTIME INTRUSIONS

No matter how carefully you have positioned your circadian rhythms to adapt to night shift work, you won't be able to sleep well in a light, noisy environment. You should invest in blackout curtains for your bedroom. When you get ready for bed, turn off your cell phone and hook up your home phone to a silent answering machine. You may also want to mask out environmental noises with a fan or a white-noise generator. Although you may find it difficult to climb into bed the minute you arrive home, try to limit your wind-down period to about one hour, and be sure you are engaging in proper "buffer period" activities such as listening to music or quiet conversation during this time.

• • •

The Insomnia Answers presented in this chapter, addressing the various ways in which your sleep might be broken, should bring you all to the very threshold of a restored state. Regardless of the twists and turns of your particular treatment path, once at this threshold, you will all face the same challenge: *to complete the journey, your mind must not lodge an objection.* Turn now to the next chapter. There, you will learn how to ease your mind's concerns and free yourself to sleep.

DIFFERENTIATE YOUR THERAPY—BROKEN SLEEP

Problem: Your sleep is broken by many awakenings.

Answer: Sleep Restriction Therapy: reduce your time in bed by the amount of time you have typically been spending awake at night (to a minimum of five hours in bed if necessary). Allow yourself an additional fifteen or thirty minutes in bed each subsequent week, so long as you are awake, on average, less than forty-five minutes each night.

Answer: Exercise four to six hours before bedtime.

Answer: Take a hot bath about three hours before bedtime.

Answer: Use Guided Imagery to shepherd your thoughts to a peaceful place.

Problem: Your sleep is scattered around the clock.

Answer: Reserve time for wakefulness instead of sleep. Establish a couple "wakeful zones" in your day, and progressively lengthen these daytime periods spent out of bed.

Problem: You awaken about every ninety minutes.

Answer: Screen for REM Sleep Disordered Breathing.

Answer: Review your use of alcohol and medications.

Answer: Calm your dreams with Imagery Rehearsal Therapy.

Problem: You work a variable shift.

Answer: Anchor Sleep: establish a base sleep period of at least four hours, obtained during the same time of day (or night) as often as possible. Fill in naps around work shifts as needed.

Problem: You work a night shift.

Answer: Wear dark or blue-blocking sunglasses in the morning.

Answer: Nap before your night shift.

Answer: Obtain bright light exposure at work.

Answer: Protect your sleep from daytime intrusions.

CHAPTER NINE

Easing Into Sleep:

Freeing Yourself to Catch the Wave

Stephanie tried not to focus on the streetlight filtering between the blinds. She played back the events one by one. Only a week or two before, she had been surrounded by a familiar group of credit analysts, paralegals, and mortgage underwriters at the large bank where she worked. (At least she had thought it was a large bank until it was swallowed whole!) Stephanie turned to rearrange the blanket, and despite herself, made out "2:39" on the digital alarm. She couldn't count many particularly close friends in her department, but it had been a comfortable place to work. She certainly didn't have to prove herself after eight years. "I'll keep my eyes closed, and pile the comforter up over here, so I can't even see the window" she thought. Mike's snoring was beginning to swell, so she straight-armed him back into a mild rasp.

Senior managers had spoken of "synergies" and "economies of scale." Yet when the merger finally took place, all Stephanie could think of was "isolation." In her new workplace, she was lost in a maze of empty cubicles, with barren partition walls and dead ends formed by stacks of hastily packed boxes. The move coordinator pointed at cartons and barked destinations, his eyes glued to his palmtop. The new boss, brought in from the other side, seemed to have taken an instant dislike to her. Even though Stephanie had been spared for the time being, she felt demoted. She was once again a trainee, with tentative sleep to match. *How appropriate,* she thought, as she flipped her pillow over to the cool side. *What a perfect way to celebrate my survival. I wonder how I'll sleep when I actually lose my job!*

No amount of pillow and blanket rearrangement will coax sleep into making an appearance when your mind is not yet fully in bed. Bewilderingly, you find yourself in two places at once: one is your bedroom in the middle of the night; the other could be just about anywhere. As with Stephanie, you might be trapped at the office. You could just as well be dwelling on medical problems, anticipating an upcoming party, fretting over a refinancing, or rehashing an argument that took place over dinner.

Initially, as you wrestle with the evening's crisis, your lack of sleep is of secondary concern. However, after several hours pass and you realize that yet another night has been squandered, the issue of sleeplessness looms larger. Eventually, the problems that earlier seemed so pressing are reduced to mere triggers. It is insomnia that packs the punch. Fidgeting in your bed, you confront the obvious fact that you are nowhere near falling asleep. Your mind is racing—thoughts and images pirouette by in a whirl. You begin to feel anxious not so much about what you are thinking, but about *how* you are thinking. At this point, you would gladly bear the steady vexation your worries brought at the beginning of the night, if only you could be relieved of the vertigo that has followed in their wake.

How can you possibly get to sleep from such a frenzied starting point? Amazingly, you usually do manage to traverse this great distance, however gracelessly. In a typical scenario, you might stay in bed tossing and turning for half the night before finally dropping off. Other times you conk out from sheer exhaustion, only to bolt upright an hour or two later. Wide awake, you give up on the whole idea of sleeping, and instead pace the floors, surf the net, or cycle through cable channels before you finally climb back into bed toward morning.

Although these responses must certainly be counted as succumbing to insomnia, they could, with just a couple modifications, be made more bearable. In contrast to the first scenario described earlier, suppose you were able to relax in bed, mind adrift, for thirty to forty-five minutes before being pulled down by a tide of drowsiness. While hardly qualifying as a great sleep onset, this experience would not be particularly wrenching either. Similarly, you could probably live with getting out of bed and reading for half an hour once or even twice to press some imaginary "reset" button, if you found yourself awake in the middle of the night. These in fact are outcomes that might result from application of two of the standard behavioral treatments for insomnia we have been discussing—Sleep Restriction Therapy and Stimulus Control Instructions. The main factor determining which way your night will fall—whether your experience will be agonizing or tolerable—is your state of mind.

The Threshold of Sleep

We start our discussion of how to put your mind at ease by positing a fundamental premise: all routes leading toward sleep, whether long or short, direct or tortuous, converge on a common threshold. This

214

jumping-off point for sleep is a place of disengagement, of indifference, and of surrender. By the time you have reached this portal, your consciousness is barely able to register its attributes. Like a basement light switch that is never seen in the "off" position because it is then too dark, the transition into sleep escapes our notice nightly.

By contrast, expulsion from the border of sleep back into full wakefulness is painfully familiar. It occurs in a flash, as the understanding that "I am not going to be able to sleep tonight" crystallizes. This realization rekindles a beam of consciousness and directs it inward, transforming what had been an increasingly shadowy mindscape into a bright mental dome filled with stark thoughts. Awareness becomes acute. We key into our anxieties and fears and become more cognizant as well of our restless bodies, surrounded by scratchy blankets, snoring bed partners, and stuffy air.

Having repeatedly experienced such abrupt ejection from the brink of sleep on account of mere thoughts, many people with insomnia understandably grow wary of their own minds. Thinking is labeled the enemy of sleep. The poor sleeper will bemoan the loss of "a switch in my brain" that was formerly available to "turn off my mind." To the chronically poor sleeper, the mind's sensitivity to the slightest jolt, its nimbleness, is a cause for alarm. Most would, therefore, be quite skeptical of our claim that this same responsiveness can be channeled in the service of sleep.

In fact, the mind's ability to give sleep the "green light" is demonstrated on an almost nightly basis: apart from those extreme cases when we literally succumb to sleep, such as after prolonged wakefulness or heavy medication, sleep is usually the result of a decision. The mind, *responding* to sleepiness, fatigue, recumbence, safety, darkness, disinterest, calm, and other favorable conditions, *permits* sleep to occur. The transaction may involve a withdrawal of interest from the external world, but it remains a choice—one that can be withdrawn at will, as insomniacs are all too aware.

How does one make a conscious choice to become unresponsive? The paradoxical ability to actively disengage might seem to be the special province of Eastern mystics, clearly out of reach of the lay insomniac. And in fact, there are commonalities between the self-hypnotic strategies and relaxation exercises that aim to bring about sleep and meditation techniques derived from Eastern philosophies. However, sleep is not enlightenment. It is not an all-or-nothing proposition, and it doesn't require perfection. Sleep can be achieved by degrees. One of sleep's more accessible way-stations, so often underappreciated by those in dire need of its comforts, is the state known as rest.

Learn to Enjoy Your Rest

If valued at all, rest is seen as a consolation prize. "I'm just resting" in the context of insomnia is a stand-in for "I'm not able to sleep." Some poor sleepers will remain in bed for hours at a time, resigned to sleeplessness, but able to at least garner the advantages of lying down, closing their eyes, and resting. However, many insomnia sufferers cannot collect even these limited benefits. When unable to sleep, these weary souls have no respite; for them, there is no middle ground between blissful sleep and torment.

If you count yourself among these unfortunates, it is time to lower your aim. Leave off your quest for sleep, and learn to rest instead. There are several reasons why this strategy makes sense. Foremost, rest is much less finicky and skittish than sleep. While it's true that in your present circumstances restfulness may seem nearly as elusive as sleep, it can in fact be pinned down. You can learn to reliably elicit a restful state. Second, while rest is not as restorative as sleep, it will have a much more refreshing effect than the hours you are currently wasting in muscle-clenching, mind-racing agitation. Third (although it is perhaps unhelpful to dwell too much on this point), restfulness can bring you to the brink of sleep. If you find your way to rest, sleep may well find you.

As noted earlier, by the time we are at the threshold of sleep, our faculties are too diminished to appreciate its contours. The same does not hold for restfulness. Our minds may not be especially acute in this state, but they are certainly capable of registering the broad outlines of both our internal state and external environment. We are able to judge for ourselves whether or not we are resting.

When speaking in physical terms, the defining feature of an object "at rest" is that it is not moving. However, it is hopefully clear to you by now that objects that think are a bit trickier to deal with. When considering a person trying to sleep, being "at rest" means not only being motionless, but also *not feeling like moving.* Sure, you could affix yourself to bed, determined not to budge an inch, but this exercise would hardly qualify as restful. Within a few moments, you would likely need to scratch an ankle, or your back would start acting up, or the blankets would feel too warm. A quick adjustment might help for a while before a new irritation arises. In short order, you would have begun the familiar "toss and turn" cycle that occupies such a large portion of an insomniac's bedtime.

In contrast to this futile chasing after immobility, think to the times when you truly did not care to move. It may have been after a long day of arduous physical toil. As you finally lay yourself down— every bone, muscle, and joint aching—you probably could not fall asleep right away, but nor did you care to. What you were really after at that moment was repose, not sleep. Whatever the position in which your body had come to rest was fine with you. You were not going to move again for quite a while, if you could help it.

The same process of disengagement can occur after a mentally taxing day. It is not surprising that after hours of intense concentration or hectic problem-solving at work, many people enjoy sitting passively in front of a television set. They have no interest in directing their attention and are only too glad to have a preassembled train of thought dispatched their way. Others may eschew the television but stare off into space with a similarly glazed demeanor, content to let their minds drift.

This is the cognitive stance that is compatible with restfulness. Just as we don't care to budge our bodies, we are not interested in pushing our thoughts in any particular direction. Instead, we follow them where they lead, slouched in a mental theater. We acknowledge the dreamlike quality of this waking state when we speak of "reveries" or "daydreams." Our thoughts may take as starting points specific events from waking life, but by the time they have wandered their course, they are barely recognizable.

We began our discussion of rest with an idealized description, but in practice the state is not imperturbable. Just as all kinds of physical discomfort can interfere with bodily repose, psychic calm is readily shattered: worry can be just as unyielding as physical pain. Even a neutral thought can insist on attention. Sometimes we are discomfited by the turn our thoughts take when we are not actively reining them in. They can head toward conflict, toward violence, toward desires that we would be reluctant to attest to by light of day.

At other times, we simply cannot tolerate the free-form, blurry, implausible productions that result from gradual withdrawal of our editorial oversight. The chaotic nature of our thinking under these conditions can induce severe anxiety. We can begin to feel as if it is our own cohesion, and not just that of our thoughts, that is dissolving. When we catch inklings that are in any way unacceptable, we may yank ourselves back into a more focused, straight-laced cognitive state with such jarring alacrity that the offending notions are lost. All we are left with is the sense that we were just on the verge of sleep, and now, for some reason, we are once again wide awake.

Let's suppose that you heed our advice and will no longer try with all your might to sleep. Rest, you decide, will suffice as a stopgap. Still, you are plagued by your own personal combination of physical and psychic ailments. Perhaps your sciatica is acting up. Maybe your car's transmission is whining, or your company has announced a major reorganization. Perhaps you are contending with a relatively trivial irritant: you wonder, for example, if you remembered to put stamps on that bunch of letters you hastily dropped in the mail on your way home from work. In any case, you've just awoken in the middle of the night, and these unresolved problems are still sullenly hanging about, as if to make you feel guilty that you excused yourself for even a short respite. You can't help but notice that it's only a bit after 2 A.M.; you've slept for barely three hours. What should you do now?

Breathe Easy

Take a deep breath. You know that much already. In moments of heightened anxiety, your respiratory rate, like your heart rate, tends to increase. These changes are part of the "fight or flight" reaction triggered by emergencies. It's not as easy to slow down your heart once it starts pumping, but you can slow down your breathing rate just by thinking about it. Take a moment to think about it right now, as a practice exercise, and slow your breathing down.

Slow your breathing down to an unnaturally slow rate, a rate that you really have to attend to to prevent yourself from speeding up. Take each deep breath through your nostrils, hold it for about three long counts, and slowly exhale through barely open lips.

Bundle your breaths in groups of three. Keep a silent count going, and each time the third breath comes along, exhale a bit more deeply, so as to let all the air out of your lungs.

The next thing we would like you to do, as you maintain this slow, steady breathing, is to choose a simple three-word phrase. This phrase could be something like "I feel relaxed," or "Time to rest," or whatever comes to mind. It will serve as a signal. Whenever you exhale deeply, on the third breath, say this phrase silently to yourself. It's at that moment that you have an opportunity to sink one notch deeper into a more restful state.

Relax Your Muscles

When you've exhaled deeply on the third breath and silently repeated the phrase you've chosen, at that moment you will be ready to release some of the muscular tension you have been carrying around all day. You store this tension without even realizing it, in places that you wouldn't expect.

For example, there is a lot of tightness around your eyes, in your forehead. Unless you happen to develop a tic, or a knot in your brow, you may not be aware of how clenched these muscles can be. Now, on the third breath, when you exhale and say the phrase you've chosen, let the muscles around your eyes and in your brow relax. Feel the difference between the state they were in just a moment ago and a slightly more relaxed state.

We're not talking about a huge difference here. We're not expecting you to somehow reverse all the strain in your brow at once. Instead, we are asking you to feel what it's like to drop down one notch, one step toward a slightly more relaxed state. The trick is to recognize that you are heading in the right direction. Once you have that skill down pat, you can always ease into a restful state. It may take a while, but you'll get there.

And wherever you focus your attention, there will be tensed muscles just waiting to relax. For example, you are no doubt aware that you carry plenty of stress in your neck and shoulders. These are large muscles, capable of storing a lot of tension. All day long they stiffen and clench, reacting to the impact of stressful events. Without some intervention, you will carry these tightened muscles right into bed with you—in fact, right into sleep.

We tend to think of sleep as the ultimate tranquil state, devoid of muscle tension. Yet falling asleep is no assurance of relaxation, as those who grind their teeth or suffer nocturnal leg cramping will sorely attest. Slow Wave Sleep, if you are lucky enough to sink to it, is associated with more relaxed muscles, while in REM sleep we lose virtually all our muscle tone. However, these sleep stages do not make up the bulk of the insomniac's sleep. In the lighter sleep stages, or when sleep is constantly interrupted by brief arousals, there is plenty of opportunity for muscular tension to impinge on restfulness. By the time you've fallen asleep, it is too late to properly relax. The tension brought forward from the day will lie in wait, ready to disrupt your night when it gets its chance.

So now, on the third breath, as you exhale and silently repeat your signal phrase, let the muscles of your neck and shoulders ease. If you're sitting up, let your head bob gently upon your shoulders. Let the cushions of the chair, or if you're already in bed, the mattress and springs, do the work of holding you up. Let yourself sink down. It feels good not to want to move at all, to be content to stay just how you are.

If you are distracted and forget to say your signal phrase as you exhale on the third breath, missing the opportunity to relax a bit more deeply, there is no need to fret. You will just hover at the level of restfulness you have already attained until the third breath returns. It's like trying to find a child you've lost sight of on a crowded merry-go-round. You wouldn't go running after her. Your best strategy is to remain still, as the child is sure to come around again.

Can you recall that wonderful feeling when, at the start of a summer vacation, you finally got to lie down on the beach? Perhaps it took a whole day to arrive at your destination, and then you had to get your bags to your room; be sure everyone else was situated; and lug towels, bags, and coolers toward the water. Finally, you had the opportunity to lay yourself down. The sand was moist, and it formed an impression around you as you let yourself sink. You didn't have to hold yourself up at all; the warm sand cradled you. There was absolutely nothing that you had to do. That's the feeling we want you to revisit nightly as you lie atop your mattress.

In a given year, we are lucky if we have one restful vacation, and even then we are usually able to find just a few moments of such absolute tranquility. Fortunately, our bodies remember these moments, and they yearn for this restful state as much as our minds do. They don't need a beach on which to find repose—just the mind's blessing, its permission to let go and spend the night adrift.

So as you drop a notch on the third breath and let more of the tension ease away from your neck and your shoulders, let your body sink down into the mattress. Let the cushions do the work of holding you. You have nowhere to go, nothing to do. It feels good to let your body waft downward into a more relaxed state.

And wherever you focus your attention, there is more muscular tightness just waiting to be released. For example, your hands have been busy all day long, typing, driving, clenching, gesturing, grasping. They've been working all day long, and you haven't given them a thought. Do so now. When you've exhaled your third breath and silently voiced your chosen signal phrase, let your fingers ease. Let your hands unfurl slightly as they rest in your lap. For just a little while, they, too, have nothing to do.

Traverse your body, surveying for hidden reservoirs of stress. Learn to appreciate the slightest ratchet downward in your level of tension. As you allow stress and tension to escape, you may notice that you feel heavier, that your limbs feel water-logged. It would take a special effort to move them now, but fortunately, you are not particularly motivated to do so. It is fine with you to just stay put. It feels good not to want to move.

Ease Your Mind Inward When the World Outside Is Chaotic

In this relaxed state, you can focus your attention wherever you choose. Your mind may not be totally clear, but at least it has blinders on. You can fixate on some things while ignoring others. You can deploy a mental barrier to protect your sleep and then take up position on the more peaceful side. If the source of your sleep disruption is external, as was the case with our patient Brenda, you can create an inner refuge for restfulness and spend your nights within its quiet confines.

Brenda's family had lived in her cozy bungalow for three generations. Her grandfather had built it on a sparsely traveled two-lane road, long since rezoned, widened, and clogged with traffic. Last spring, her neighbor sold out to a large shopping mall developer. Brenda didn't have enough land to sell for commercial purposes—and now, her beloved home was pretty much worthless on the residential market.

The huge tractors didn't get underway until evening; then they cranked all night long. At sporadic intervals, they would drop thick steel plates, shaking the entire house. Brenda was assaulted, too, by the staccato shrieks issued by these vehicles as they backed up. The town board had been patronizing, noting that it was hard to build a mega-mall quietly. There was less traffic for the crews to contend with at night, they added.

After a few months, Brenda came to consider the periods of relative quiet to be more distressing than the noise. When would they end? She began to compulsively time intervals between clashes on her digital clock—eleven minutes was the record so far. Sleeping pills might provide a respite for three or four hours, but after that, Brenda emerged into a fitful half-sleep, once again at the mercy of the "progress" being made just outside her door.

What can be done for someone trapped in such circumstances? While the broader aim of therapy was to support Brenda's efforts to obtain just compensation, pull up stakes, and start afresh, in the meantime, she needed to get at least a bit more sleep. "Egg carton" sound-attenuating foam insulation and a white-noise generator abetted her sleeping pills somewhat. Her mind was able to be recruited to help in the effort as well.

With practice, Brenda learned to focus her attention away from the construction zone across the road and toward another piece of real estate. Currently located only in her mind's eye, it held out the promise of one day being quite real—for it was Brenda's dream home, the place in which she would eventually find refuge from her waking nightmare. Following slow breathing and muscle relaxation, Brenda visited this idyllic home at night. She explored its nooks and wandered its grounds. In turn, she stopped attending so scrupulously to every noise that shot across the road. Secluded in her imaginary garden, nestled between its raised beds, Brenda was better able to drift off to sleep.

There is no need to wait until the bulldozers arrive before you, too, learn how to enlist your mind's eye as a calming ally. Start building your own internal sanctuary so it will be ready if you need it. Once you have slowed down your breathing, bundled your breaths in groups of three, chosen a phrase to signal that the tension trapped within you has an opportunity to slip away—once you have achieved a restful state—allow yourself twenty minutes or so in your imagined refuge.

A good location on which to construct such a mental haven would be a vacation spot you actually visited, perhaps when you were younger and more carefree. Remember, it was during the long summer break, without homework hanging over your head. Is there a particular lakeside park, mountain meadow, or ocean beach that comes to mind? Don't be satisfied to recall just its name. Bring it to life. If there were trees, imagine them rustling in the wind. What does their bark look like? What kind of shade do they provide? Is the sun hot or the breeze cool? Is the ground rocky or soft? The more details you provide, the easier it will be to dwell in your sleep shelter. Remember, you've been there before, and both your body and your mind are longing to return. Give them a nudge in the right direction, and they will find their way back.

Focus Outward When the Turmoil Lies Within

In practice, the disruption that is most likely to intrude on sleep is not to be found across the street or in a neighboring apartment—rather, it is the distress that is carried within your mind. It can take the form of a small misgiving, a nagging worry, or a horrific memory. Regardless of its scale, internal distress is by nature difficult to uproot. It cannot be excised by sheer mental effort.

To secure relief from an internal adversary, you need to be wily. You can perform a bit of mental alchemy and change a tormenting memory into something more benign, as with the Imagery Rehearsal Therapy we discussed earlier. You can build an inner refuge, protected by a barrier that attenuates tormenting thoughts, just as Brenda was able to inure herself to construction noise. You can also learn to focus your attention outside yourself. You can train your perception on the subtleties of the external world, where there is always an innocuous parade filing by, ready to distract your mind from drifting into troublesome realms. We made recourse to all of these strategies when helping Leeann to find some peace at night.

Leeann's sleep was full of holes, and so were her bedroom walls. She was still sleeping in the same upstairs room where, nearly six years earlier, she had been jarred awake to find a knife pressed against her throat and her mother's boyfriend atop her diminutive body. With sentence reductions for good behavior, he could look forward to getting out of prison in the not too distant future. Leeann, though, was still confined by a panic that gripped her nightly.

Leeann managed to steel herself during the day. She had learned to paint enough of a smile on her face to forestall complaints from customers in the infants' wear department where she had become a fixture. She focused so intently on her precise flannel folds that buyers didn't seem to notice that she never caught their eye.

While her armor was adequate to daytime challenges, it was less reliable warding off anxiety at night. As evening fell, Leeann could sense her skin tightening and her mouth going dry. Her unease transformed into despair once she got into bed. Usually, she would just sob quietly. However, several years ago, Leeann had discovered that the fiberboard panels that made up the wainscoting around her room would yield with a satisfying crack if she punched with all her might, aiming midway between the wall studs as best as she could judge. The fact that these studs were somewhat irregularly spaced, leading occasionally to injuries more serious than a bruise, seemed to Leeann an added inducement.

In addition to working with trauma counselors early on, Leeann was taking sedating and antidepressant medications under the care of a psychiatrist, and she had a therapist whom she had seen regularly for years. She drew great comfort and support from these professionals. We were fortunate to be able to rely on and build upon her work with them—it allowed us to concentrate on her agitated nights and elusive sleep. Our task was to find zones of safety, however microscopic, in a world that had betrayed Leeann's trust.

We started by transforming, as best we could, Leeann's bedroom. Initially, she had decided that financial constraints prevented her from simply leaving this traumatic setting. We still wished to signal the start of a new era by changing its look. Leeann was encouraged to rearrange furniture, replace pictures, and buy a down comforter. She softened the lighting and strategically positioned quilts over the worst of the damaged walls.

These measures proved to be more symbolic than therapeutic. Ultimately, when a suitable apartment appeared for rent in the next town, Leeann made the leap and almost immediately she felt an increased sense of security. She no longer had to gaze at the same ceiling cracks she had fixed on during the rape. She no longer was reminded by the raggedy punctured wainscoting of her helplessness and rage.

Even in her new home, however, Leeann felt that the night was not to be trusted. The dark world outside her windows contained too many unknowns, too many potential threats. Threats of another sort also lurked within the recesses of her mind, ready to spring if she allowed her thoughts to stray too close. We made an agreement that bedtime was not the time to deal with either of these adversaries. The best place for Leeann's attention to alight, for her to find respite, was on the easily overlooked buffer between the inner and outer worlds. She learned to focus on the physical sensations that enveloped her as she lay in bed, snug in her new comforter.

There is so much going on about you on a sensory level that you would quickly be overwhelmed if you attended to it all. Fortunately, your brain is adept at filtering out nearly all this extraneous stimulation. You don't notice every waft of air that comes your way. Instead, you save your reaction for the cold draft that gives you goose bumps. You don't pay any mind to furnaces cranking up, footsteps squeaking on tiled floors, or muffled voices down the hall. These sounds all blend comfortably into a background drone, leaving you free to concentrate on the task at hand until a major intrusion such as a blasting car horn grabs your attention. This filtering is a good thing, allowing us to function more efficiently when we are awake, as well as preserving our sleep. However, when we are caught at the border of sleep, unable to pass through, it is helpful to turn off this filtering feature and open ourselves to all the tiny intrusions that come our way.

Train yourself to become more sensitive to slight variations in the temperature of your bedroom and to the way that air movements distribute these differences. Focus on these air currents as they brush past the skin of your face, hands, and arms. If it is a cold winter night, try to feel the coolness that congregates by the window. If a radiator is on, take a few moments to sense the heat reaching to you from across the room, or the warm air convections that have been set in motion. If on a crisp fall night you have cracked open the window, feel the refreshing surge that is admitted into your bedroom each time a breeze kicks up.

Attend to the slightest of sounds. As you lie in bed, become more attuned to the distant sound of traffic, the slurp of your dog licking its paw, the various pings and creaks your house emits while cooling off from a day in the sun. Yes, there is a fatigue that sets in after a while—it's difficult to stay so focused. Just listen to what you can. As brief dips into sleep temporarily shut down your perception, you will inevitably miss out on many sounds. That's all right. They'll be there if you need them again.

Finally, don't overlook the sense of touch. If you are feeling cool, allow a blanket to drape your skin, bringing not only warmth but a comforting sense of enclosure. Focus on the gentle contact made, on the slight pressure exerted by the fabric. The same cocooned feeling can be achieved with a fresh sheet in warmer seasons. If you've been banished from bed because your tossing and turning disturbed a bed partner, perhaps you can gain readmission if you demonstrate that you have finally learned how to rest. Snuggling together, take a silent survey of how many places your bodies are touching. If it is too warm for such closeness, all your tactile focus can be channeled into

229

the contact made through one hand. Synchronize your breathing, and sense the rhythmic rise and fall of the blankets that ensue. Such purely physical sensations are blessedly neutral, safely distracting your mind while sleep makes its approach.

Suspended in a state of rest, you are content to let your mind and body ease. This relaxed state is not sleep, but it has its own rewards. Your muscles are grateful for their stillness; your thoughts appreciate their freedom from scrutiny. You can comfortably disregard the demands of the external world, at least until tomorrow. You can refuse to entertain worries for the night, cordoning them off to the side of consciousness. You imagine the plentiful supply of sleep drive you providently stored across the previous day, more than sufficient to fuel sleep through the night. You picture yourself easing down the circadian slope of alertness, so carefully groomed by all the actions you have taken in recent weeks. You are ready to sleep, but you are already at rest. The night will be good.

One-Month Check-Up

The Insomnia Answer is designed to produce rapid results. Our Preliminary Treatment is intended to remove obstacles to better sleep, strengthen your homeostatic Sleep Drive, and synchronize your sleep/wake schedule with internal circadian rhythms so your time in bed is more likely to be filled with deep sleep. All these benefits should accrue regardless of the nature of your sleep problem. Targeted treatments should then further improve your sleep where it has been most disrupted. It is now time to take stock of your gains and see what more needs to be done. Once again, we will ask you to fill out the Insomnia Symptom Questionnaire and the Fatigue Severity Scale.

INSOMNIA SYMPTOM QUESTIONNAIRE

NEVER	N
RARELY	R
SOMETIMES	S
FREQUENTLY	F
ALWAYS	A

Patient: _____

Day: _____ Date: _____ Time: _____

Answer the following questions based on the <u>previous 7 days</u>.

1. Do you lie awake at night worried, anxious or distressed? N R S F A

2. During the day do you worry about how you will sleep that night? N R S F A

3. Are you watching the clock or aware of time passing while lying awake in bed? N R S F A

4. Is your sleep restless? N R S F A

5. Are you experiencing <u>brief</u> awakenings during the night? N R S F A

6. Are you experiencing <u>long</u> awakenings during the night? N R S F A

7. Do you feel tired or fatigued during the day or evening? N R S F A

8. Have you taken any naps or fallen asleep briefly during the day or evening? N R S F A

9. Have you been sleepy or drowsy during the day or evening? N R S F A

10. Do you feel you have been getting an adequate amount of sleep? N R S F A

11. Do you feel you have been getting good quality sleep? N R S F A

12. Since the last time you answered this questionnaire is your sleep now . . .
    Much Better   Better   No Different   Worse   Much Worse

Afterword

FATIGUE SEVERITY SCALE

This scale contains nine statements relating to fatigue and its consequences. Read each statement and circle a number from 1 to 7, depending on how well you feel the statement applies to you, judging from the preceding week. A low value indicates that the statement hardly applies to you, whereas a high value indicates that the statement applies very well.

During the past week, I have found that: **Score**

1. My motivation is lower when I am fatigued.   1 2 3 4 5 6 7

2. Exercise brings on my fatigue.   1 2 3 4 5 6 7

3. I am easily fatigued.   1 2 3 4 5 6 7

4. Fatigue interferes with my physical functioning.   1 2 3 4 5 6 7

5. Fatigue causes frequent problems for me.   1 2 3 4 5 6 7

6. My fatigue prevents sustained physical functioning.   1 2 3 4 5 6 7

7. Fatigue interferes with carrying out certain duties and responsibilities.   1 2 3 4 5 6 7

8. Fatigue is among my three most disabling symptoms. 1 2 3 4 5 6 7

9. Fatigue interferes with my work, family, or social life. 1 2 3 4 5 6 7

Score by calculating the average response to the questions (adding up all the answers and dividing by nine).

Your Sleep and Fatigue Are Much Improved

If you rate your Insomnia Symptoms and Fatigue as having substantially diminished, we suggest continuing all treatment strategies without change for another month. This will consolidate your gains and make your sleep even more robust. Most of you veteran insomniacs have experienced periods of inexplicably better sleep for a few weeks, only to relapse into another flare-up. It will take time to gain confidence that lasting change has actually taken place. As nights of reasonably good sleep accumulate, you will begin to pay less attention to the whole issue. Inevitable night-to-night variations in sleep quantity or quality will be incorporated into your expectations and balance out each other, prompting no need for corrective action.

Your Sleep Has Improved but Your Fatigue Has Not

Many of the treatments presented in *The Insomnia Answer* are likely to increase fatigue at least initially. With improving sleep quality, better circadian regulation, and gradually increasing time spent asleep, this fatigue should diminish. However, if your sleep has improved substantially while fatigue remains a problem, you should consider the possibility that this fatigue is due to another sleep disorder or has origins outside of the sleep/wake system. You should consult your physician regarding such persistent fatigue as a full diagnostic work-up may be required, considering many organ systems and diseases. With regards to other sleep disturbances, an evaluation at a Sleep Disorder Center may be advised to assess for

Obstructive Sleep Apnea, Narcolepsy, Restless Legs Syndrome, Periodic Limb Movements, or other conditions associated with sleepiness or fatigue.

Your Sleep Has Not Improved

What if there has been no improvement in your insomnia symptoms? First, check that you have complied with *all* our recommendations. In their desperation, many poor sleepers will run through a series of interventions, abandoning those that appear to have no effect. They will forego all caffeine for two weeks, for example, but resume drinking coffee just as they try eliminating their afternoon naps. While this strategy may sound like a reasonable effort to isolate the "cause" of the problem, our 3P Model emphasizes the compound nature of sleeplessness: insomnia often arises from the confluence of many factors, and you may have to simultaneously redress a host of these, large and small, to gain traction.

Therefore, it behooves you to review the ABCs of the Insomnia Answer and diligently follow all its preliminary recommendations before you apply more specific treatments. Then, if your treatment path has not already introduced a full-strength application of Sleep Restriction Therapy (cutting out *all* extra wakefulness from your bedtime schedule rather than just half of it), you should apply this treatment, discussed in Chapter 8. Similarly, if you are continuing to experience prolonged nocturnal awakenings and have not yet followed Stimulus Control Instructions (appearing in Chapters 6 and 7), now is the time to do so. In conjunction with these interventions, we advise that you not allow yourself even one hour of oversleeping on weekends, but instead get up at the same time seven days a week.

If you have put all recommended treatment interventions in place, have strictly limited "exceptions to the rule," are not facing any life crises that may require direct psychotherapeutic or psychiatric intervention, and are still not seeing much progress, two potential culprits come to mind: continuing hyperarousal, which should be countered in a straightforward manner, and self-sabotage, which is a more wily adversary.

In the case of hyperarousal, redouble your efforts to exercise regularly (preferably in the late afternoon) and increase the intensity of your workout. In addition, be consistent in setting aside time for Guided Imagery. Like any skill, this cognitive therapy improves with practice, and the arousal-dampening effect you can achieve after one month hardly hints at its full potential. If these measures fall short, consider a brief trial on a hypnotic medication to supplement your cognitive-behavioral treatment. Studies have shown that the combination of approaches is quite effective.

Self-sabotage sounds quite nefarious. We're sure there are some instances where sleeplessness is a chosen means of self-destruction, but more typically it is fear, anxiety, or perhaps just skepticism that leads people to sabotage their own sleep. In the opening chapters of this book, we emphasized how sleep is uniquely susceptible to disturbance merely by thinking. People who have discovered this through hard experience are understandably jittery when it comes to trusting that sleep will show up on cue. If the thought *I don't think I'm going to sleep tonight* is still leading you to that very result, you may well feel doomed to sleeplessness.

In this case, we have some advice that may be surprising: don't follow our program so closely. We're not suggesting that you abandon it totally, but back off a bit, in enough ways to enable you to get on with your life without feeling too constrained. For example, don't resume drinking your usual six cups of coffee, but hold yourself to one or two in the morning. You don't have to strictly limit yourself anymore to five hours of bedtime, but see if you can live with seven and a half, scheduled around the hours you are most likely to sleep, rather than sleeping as catch can. Don't worry about getting every minute of your suggested bright light exposure every day, but get as much as possible.

Once you've made such adjustments, let time take over the therapy. You will need at least a few more months to convince yourself that any progress is possible. Just as with the lovelorn example met up with in our preface, healing will sneak up on you when you least expect it. You may not notice much difference night to night, but over time, you will see that the intensity of your insomnia has at least diminished somewhat. This minor victory will allow you to return to our full program in the future with increased confidence, and meet with greater success.

CHAPTER 1

(a) *A review article that presents a comprehensive review of theoretical issues in insomnia.*

Espie, CA. "Insomnia: Conceptual Issues in the Development, Persistence, and Treatment of Sleep Disorder in Adults." *Annual Review of Psychology*, 2002; 53: 215–243.

(b) *Insomnia has wide-ranging effects on insomnia sufferers as illustrated in this article.*

Zammit, GK, Weiner, J, Damato, N, Sillup, GP, McMillan, CA. "Quality of life in people with insomnia." *Sleep*, 1999; 22 (Suppl 2): S379–385.

CHAPTER 2

(a) *This paper presents one of the earliest models of homeostatic and circadian influences on sleep regulation.*

Borbely, AA. "A two process model of sleep regulation." *Hum Neurobiol.*, 1982; 1(3):195–204.

(b) *A well-controlled study showing that one cycle of the biological clock is very close to twenty-four hours.*

Czeisler, CA, Duffy, JF, Shanahan, TL, Brown, EN, Mitchell, JF, Rimmer, DW, Ronda, JM, Silva, EJ, Allan, JS, Emens, JS, Dijk, DJ, Kronauer, RE. "Stability, precision, and near-24-hour period of the human circadian pacemaker." *Science*, 1999; 284(5423):2177–2181.

(c) *This paper presents an elegant model of the neural mechanisms that regulate sleep and wakefulness. It details the process by which these two states are triggered and switched.*

Clifford, B. Saper, Thomas C. Chou, and Thomas E. Scammell. "The sleep switch: hypothalamic control of sleep and wakefulness." *Trends in Neurosciences,* Vol. 24, Issue 12, December 1, 2001, p. 726–731.

Available by download at http://www.sciencedirect.com/science?. The digital object identifier is doi:10.1016/S0166-2236(00)02002-6.

(d) *The interaction of the circadian and the homeostatic systems is discussed in this journal publication.*

Edgar, Dale M., Dement, William C., and Fuller, Charles A. "Effect of SCN Lesions on Sleep in Squirrel Monkeys: Evidence for Opponent Processes in Sleep-Wake Regulation." *The Journal of Neuroscience,* March 1993, 13(3): 1065–1079.

Available by download at http://www.jneurosci.org/cgi/reprint/13/3/1065.

CHAPTER 3

(a) *One of the original articles describing the authors' 3P Model of Insomnia (Predisposing, Precipitating, and Perpetuating factors) with a graphic depiction. Figures 14 and 16 are adapted from this article. The current version of our model has been much improved with the help of Dr. Max Hirshkowitz.*

Spielman, AJ, Caruso, L, and Glovinsky, P. "A behavioral perspective on insomnia treatment." *Psychiatric Clinics of North America,* 1987; 10(4): 541–553.

(b) *A series of chapters that review the models of insomnia and a variety of treatments. All are in MH Kryger, T Roth, and WC Dement (eds). Principles and Practice of Sleep Medicine, Fourth Edition. Philadelphia, Elsevier Saunders, 2005.*

1. Perlis, ML, Smith, MT, and Pigeon, WR. "Etiology and Pathophysiology of Insomnia." 714–725.
2. Morin, CM. "Psychological and Behavioral Treatments for Primary Insomnia." 726–737.
3. Lichstein, KL, Nau, SD, McCrae, CS, and Stone, KC. "Psychological and Behavioral Treatments for Secondary Insomnias." 738–748.
4. Walsh, JT, Roehrs, T, and Roth, T. "Pharmacological Treatment of Primary Insomnia." 749–760.
5. Spielman, AJ, Yang, CM, and Glovinsky, PG. "Assessment Techniques for Insomnia." 1403–1416.
6. Buysse, DJ, Schweitzer, PK, and Moul, DE. "Clinical Pharmacology of Other Drugs Used as Hypnotics." 452–467.

(c) *Articles that identify physiological bases for hyperarousal in insomnia.*

Perlis, ML, Kehr, EL Smith, MT, Andrews, PJ, Orff, H, and Giles, DE. "Temporal and stagewise distribution of high frequency EEG activity in patients with primary and secondary insomnia and in good sleeper controls." *Journal of Sleep Research*, 2001; 10(2): 93–104.

Bonnet, MH, Arand, DL. "24-Hour metabolic rate in insomniacs and matched normal sleepers." *Sleep*, 1995; 581–588.

(d) *This study shows increased alertness in insomnia supporting the hyperarousal model.*

Stepanski, E, Zorick, F, Roehrs, T, Young, D, Roth, T. "Daytime alertness in patients with chronic insomnia compared with asymptomatic control subjects." *Sleep*, 1988; 11(1):54–60.

(e) *This study shows that caffeine ingestion in the morning is not without its effects on brain waves at night.*

Landolt, HP, Werth, E, Borbely, AA, Dijk, DJ. "Caffeine intake (200 mg) in the morning affects human sleep and EEG power spectra at night." *Brain Res.*, 1995; 675(1–2):67–74.

CHAPTER 4

(a) *A discussion of the ways in which our minds can sabotage our sleep.*

Harvey, AG. "Trouble in bed: The role of pre-sleep worry and intrusion in the maintenance of insomnia." *Journal of Cognitive Psychotherapy: An International Quarterly*, 2002; 16:161–177.

CHAPTER 5

(a) *Current diagnostic criteria established for research in insomnia.*

Edinger, JD, Bonnet, MH, Bootzin, RR, Doghramji, K, Dorsey, CM, Espie, CA, Jamieson, AO, McCall, WV, Morin, CM, Stepanski, EJ. "Derivation of research diagnostic criteria for insomnia: report of an American Academy of Sleep Medicine work group." *Sleep*, 2004; 27:1567–1596.

(b) *The Insomnia Symptom Questionnaire was first published in our initial paper on Sleep Restriction (listed here under Chapter 8).*

Questions 1–3 relate to worry about sleep. Trouble sleeping is covered in questions 4–6. The daytime consequences of sleep loss are rated in questions 7–9. Questions 10–12 ask for global assessments of how your sleep has changed. In general, people with insomnia tend to indicate that symptoms on the Insomnia

Symptom Questionnaire appear Frequently or Always. However, the manifestations of insomnia vary greatly between individuals. Therefore, you need not compare your scores on this questionnaire with typical scores. It is more important to assess whether *your* symptom frequency is reduced after treatment.

(c) *The source of the Fatigue Severity Scale.*

Krupp LB, LaRocca NG, Muir-Nash J, Steinberg AD. "The Fatigue Severity Scale: Application to Patients with Multiple Sclerosis and Systemic Lupus Erythematosus." *Archives of Neurology*, 1989; 46, 1121–1123.

Add up the ratings you selected for each item to obtain a total score. There is no cutoff score on this scale that identifies a person as having insomnia. In fact, fatigue is a common symptom of many medical and psychological disorders. The Fatigue Severity Scale's main use is to compare levels of fatigue before and after treatment. Note that some behavioral treatments for insomnia may initially increase your fatigue level, but fatigue should subside as sleep becomes more consolidated.

(d) *The source of the Sleep Hygiene Awareness and Practices Questionnaire.* The first fifteen items indicate practices that may interfere with building a robust sleep-wake cycle. For the sake of consistency, we have modified items 4, 6, and 7. The final four items are recommended to help sleep.

Lacks P. *Behavioral Treatment for Persistent Insomnia.* New York: Pergamon Press, 1987.

(e) *A concise review of good sleep hygiene practices.*

Hauri PJ. *The Sleep Disorders.* Current Concepts second ed. Kalamazoo, Michigan: Upjohn, 1982.

(f) *The source of the Zung Depression Rating Scale.*

Zung, WWK, "A self-rating depression scale." *Arch Gen Psychiatry*, 1965; 12:63–70.

The scoring of the Zung Self-Rating Depression Scale requires you to assign a value to each response and then add up these ratings. Your responses are scored one way for half of the questions; the values are then reversed for the other questions, as follows:

Responses	Values for Questions 1, 3, 4, 7, 8, 9, 10, 13, 15, 19	Values for Questions 2, 5, 6, 11, 12, 14, 16, 17, 18, 20
"A little of the time"	1	4
"Some of the time"	2	3

"Good part of the time"	3	2
"Most of the time"	4	1

A total score of 50 to 59 suggests a minimal to mild depression, while a score of 60 to 69 represents a moderate to marked depression, and a 70 or more suggests a severe to extreme depression.

(g) *The source of the Pre-Sleep Arousal Scale.*

Nicassio, PM, Mendlowitz, DR, Fussell, JJ, et al. "The phenomenology of the pre-sleep state: the development of the pre-sleep arousal scale." *Behav Res Ther.,* 1985; 23:263–271.

The Pre-sleep Arousal Scale assesses two areas—physiological hyperarousal (item numbers 1, 2, 5, 7, 10, 12, 13, and 15) and cognitive hyperarousal (item numbers 3, 4, 6, 8, 9, 11, 14, and 16). Individuals with insomnia average about 2 (a little) on the physiological items and 3 (moderate) on the cognitive items. However, we caution against relying on a single score to assess the degree to which hyperarousal is playing a role in *your* sleep disturbance. This scale is best used to focus attention on the particular cognitive or physiological aspects of hyperarousal you need to address.

(h) *The source of the Dysfunctional Beliefs and Attitudes about Sleep scale. The version presented here is a shortened form used by Dr. Morin.*

Morin, CM: *Insomnia: Psychological Assessment and Management.* New York: The Guilford Press, 1993.

People with insomnia tend to mark the lines on this scale somewhere on the half indicating stronger agreement with each statement. Note that item 23 is the exception; marks indicating *disagreement* with this statement are associated with insomnia.

(i) *An early article on the brain wave changes that are produced by a warm bath in the evening.*

Horne, JA, Reid, AJ. "Night-time sleep EEG changes following body heating in a warm bath." *Electroencephalogr Clin Neurophysiol.* 1985; 60(2): 154–157.

CHAPTER 6

(a) *This article is a well-controlled study of the effects of varying the timing of light exposure on the timing of circadian rhythms.*

Sat Bir S. Khalsa, Megan E. Jewett, Christian Cajochen, and Charles A. Czeisler. "A phase response curve to single bright light pulses in human subjects." *J Physiol.,* 2003; 549.3:945–952.

Download available at http://jp.physoc.org/cgi/content/full/549/3/945.

Endnotes

(b) *This study establishes a method of assessing the level of subjective sleepiness that corresponds to readiness for sleep.*

Yang, CM., Lin, FW, and Spielman, AJ. "Standard instructions for the evaluation of subjective sleepiness: A validation study." *Sleep*, 2004; 27(2):329–332.

(c) *A description of how to conduct treatment using Stimulus Control Instructions.*

Bootzin, RR, Epstein, D, Wood, JM. "Stimulus Control Instructions." In Hauri, P (ed). *Case studies in insomnia.* New York; Plenum Press, 1991, 19–28.

(d) *A study that demonstrates that putting subjects in the dark before bedtime shifts sleep to an earlier time, with implications for the treatment of sleep-onset insomnia.*

Van Cauter, E. Moreno-Reyes, R, Akseki, E, L'Hermite-Balériaux, M, Hirschfeld, U, Leproult, R, Copinschi, G. "Rapid phase advance of the 24-h melatonin profile in response to afternoon dark exposure." *Am J Physiol Endocrinol Metab*, 1998; 275: E48-E54.

Download available at http://ajpendo.physiology.org/cgi/content/full/275/1/E48.

(e) *The first study that systematically showed taking melatonin supplementation shifts circadian rhythms in a predictable manner.*

Lewy AJ, Ahmed S, Jackson JML et al. "Melatonin shifts human circadian rhythms according to a phase-response curve." *Chronobiology International*, 1992; 9:380–392.

(f) *The first study that defined the delayed sleep phase disorder and offered an effective treatment.*

Weitzman, E. D., Czeisler, C., Coleman, R., Spielman, A. J., Zimmerman, J., Dement, W. C., Richardson, G., and Pollak, C. P. "Delayed sleep phase syndrome: A chronobiological disorder with sleep onset insomnia." *Archives of General Psychiatry*, 1981; 38:737–746.

(g) *This article focuses on clinical manifestations of sleep phase delay in adolescents.*

Thorpy, M. J., Korman, E., Spielman, A. J., and Glovinsky, P. B. "Delayed sleep phase syndrome in adolescents." *Journal of Adolescent Health Care*, 1988; 9: 22–27.

(h) *A report describing treatment of delayed sleep phase disorder by delivering bright light through the closed eyelids of sleeping patients.*

Cole RJ, Smith JS, Alcala YC, Elliot JA, Kripke DF. "Bright-light mask treatment of delayed sleep phase syndrome." *J. Biol. Rhythms*, 2002; 17(1): 89–101.

Endnotes

CHAPTER 7

(a) *These two articles present research showing that bright light exposure in the evening addresses difficulty maintaining sleep.*

Campbell, S, Dawson, D, Anderson, MW. "Alleviation of sleep maintenance insomnia with timed exposure to bright light." *Journal of American Geriatric Society*, 1993; 4:829–836.

L. Lack, H. Wright, S., Gibbon, and E. Kempth. "The treatment of early morning awakening insomnia with 2 evenings of bright light." *Sleep*, 2005; 28(5): 616–623.

(b) *A report that summarizes a number of studies showing the effectiveness of cognitive behavioral therapy compared to hypnotic medications for insomnia.*

Michael T. Smith, Michael L. Perlis, Amy Park, Michelle S. Smith, JaeMi Pennington, Donna E. Giles, and Daniel J. Buysse. "Comparative Meta-Analysis of Pharmacotherapy and Behavior Therapy for Persistent Insomnia." *Am. J. Psychiatry*, 2002; 159:5–11.

Download available at http://ajp.psychiatryonline.org/cgi/content/full/159/ 1/5.

CHAPTER 8

(a) *The original article presenting Sleep Restriction Therapy.*

Spielman AJ, Saskin P, Thorpy MJ. "Treatment of chronic insomnia by restriction of time in bed." *Sleep*, 1987; 10:45–56.

Our original method of administering Sleep Restriction Therapy was a bit more complicated and allowed for both additions and subtractions to bedtime each week. As with the method described here, we started by assigning time in bed equal to each patient's average nightly sleep time estimated from a two-week Sleep Log. Then the patient's sleep efficiency during the first week on the restricted bedtime schedule was calculated by dividing that week's average sleep time by the length of the assigned bedtime. If this sleep efficiency was 90 percent or greater, bedtime would be extended by fifteen minutes. If it was 85 percent or less, bedtime would be shortened by fifteen minutes. If sleep efficiency was between 85 percent and 90 percent, no change in bedtime length would be made for that week.

Using the sample log presented in Chapter 8 to illustrate, the average amount of sleep time across the week was about 5.5 hours. Dividing this figure by 6 hours (the length of the assigned bedtime) yields a sleep efficiency of just under 92 percent. Therefore, our model insomniac would be allowed an extra 15 minutes of bedtime during the coming week.

This research version of Sleep Restriction Therapy was demonstrated to quickly improve sleep efficiency and reduce night-to-night variability in total esti-

mated sleep time. Eventually, subjects in our protocols estimated that they slept a bit longer as well, but the main benefit of the treatment appears to be that it lessens anxiety over how much sleep will occur on a given night, which in turn increases the chances that sleep will appear. We have found that we can retain these benefits of the research version of Sleep Restriction Therapy, while avoiding the potentially demoralizing effect of further reductions in bedtime, through the modification presented in this book. Once you make the initial adjustment in bedtime length, you can reasonably expect to spend more time in bed as the treatment progresses.

(b) *A way to address recurrent nightmares through scripted rehearsal of dream content with more benign endings.*

Krakow, B, Kellner, R, Pathak, D, Lambert, L. "Imagery rehearsal treatment for chronic nightmares." *Behaviour Research and Therapy*, 1995; 33(7): 837–843.

(c) *A review and two research reports relating to shift work sleep problems and how best to address them.*

Eastman, CI, Martin, SK. "How to use light and dark to produce circadian adaptation to night shift work." *Ann Med.*, 1999; 31(2): 87–98.

Fogg, LF, Eastman, CI. "Combinations of bright light, scheduled dark, sunglasses and melatonin to facilitate circadian entrainment to night shift work." *Journal of Biological Rhythms*, 2003; 18: 513–523.

Boivin, DB, James, FO. "Circadian adaptation to night-shift work by judicious light and darkness exposure." *Journal of Biological Rhythms*, 2002; 17: 556–567.

(d) *A research report describing how "anchor sleep" helps stabilize circadian rhythms in people following irregular sleep schedules.*

Minors, D, Waterhouse, J. "Anchor sleep as a synchronizer of rhythms on abnormal routines." *Int. J Chronobiology*, 1981; 7(3): 165–168.

INDEX

Index

Index

Paul Glovinsky, Ph.D., has been helping people achieve better sleep for more than twenty-five years. He is the clinical director of the Capital Region Sleep/Wake Disorders Center in Albany, New York. Dr. Glovinsky also maintains a private practice in New York City as a clinical psychologist specializing in the treatment of sleep disorders and anxiety disorders, and is an adjunct professor at The City College of the City University of New York. He is a Diplomate of the American Board of Sleep Medicine, where he has served as an insomnia specialist. He is currently the head of the Examination Committee for the Behavioral Sleep Medicine section of the American Academy of Sleep Medicine. Working with Kaplan Educational Centers, Dr. Glovinsky has consulted with educational institutions, nonprofit organizations, and Fortune 500 companies, with a focus on performance enhancement under stressful conditions. He has been featured in numerous print, radio, and television stories ranging from the treatment of sleep disorders to dealing with test anxiety.

Arthur Spielman, Ph.D., is recognized as one of the foremost experts on insomnia in the world. A clinical psychologist, Dr. Spielman has been evaluating and treating patients with sleeping difficulties for thirty years. He and his colleagues have written numerous chapters in textbooks and research reports on insomnia. He has given more than one hundred invited lectures at medical schools, universities, and hospitals. He has served as an expert on insomnia for organizations such as the National Institutes of Health, American Academy of Sleep Medicine, and American Board of Sleep Medicine. Dr. Spielman has also provided public education about sleep problems on national television, on radio, in newspapers, in magazines, and on the Internet.

Dr. Spielman was the psychologist at the first accredited sleep disorders center in the United States in 1976. Over the years, he has worked at six sleep disorders centers. He is professor of psychology at The City College of the City University of New York and associate director at the Sleep Disorder Centers at New York Methodist Hospital, Brooklyn, New York; Danbury Hospital, Danbury, Connecticut; and New York Presbyterian Hospital—Weill Medical College of Cornell University.

If you are interested in finding a behavioral sleep medicine expert certified by the American Academy of Sleep Medicine, a current listing is available at their website. The direct link is www.aasmnet.org/BSME.aspx. This credential has been issued for just a few years, so as of this writing there are only sixty-five certified specialists. More will be joining each year as training programs are developed within graduate schools and in accredited sleep centers.